SISTERS
OF THE
EAST END

SISTERS
OF THE
EAST END

The real stories of the Sisters who inspired
CALL THE MIDWIFE

HELEN BATTEN

and the Sisters of the Community of St John the Divine

EBURY
PRESS

3 5 7 9 10 8 6 4 2

First published in 2013 by Ebury Press, an imprint of Ebury Publishing
A Random House Group company

The Random House Group Limited Reg. No. 954009

Addresses for companies within the Random House Group can be found at
www.randomhouse.co.uk

A CIP catalogue record for this book is available from the British Library

The Random House Group Limited supports the Forest Stewardship
Council® (FSC®), the leading international forest certification organisation.
Our books carrying the FSC label are printed on FSC® certified paper. FSC is
the only forest certification scheme supported by the leading environmental
organisations, including Greenpeace. Our paper procurement policy can be
found at www.randomhouse.co.uk/environment

Printed and bound by CPI Group (UK) Ltd, Croydon, CR0 4YY

ISBN 9780091951771

To buy books by your favourite authors and register for offers visit
www.randomhouse.co.uk

AUTHOR'S NOTE

The story of Sister Catherine Mary has been created from interviews with the six sisters of the Community of St John the Divine. Although fictional, her life is based on the real experiences of the Sisters, particularly the Reverend Mothers Christine and Margaret Angela, and their lives working as nurses and midwives in the East End and abroad.

I first met the Sisters over a year ago and was immediately struck by their warmth, humour and love. Then, as they told me their stories, I was amazed by the history of their Community, the pioneering and largely unsung work of these courageous, feisty women who dedicated their lives to helping the poor and played such a key role in developing nursing and midwifery in this country. It made me think about the real meaning of commitment: as well as constant challenges, I learned how it brings great rewards. They have been an inspiration.

I would like to thank Sisters Christine, Margaret Angela, Theresa, Ivy, Elaine, Shirley and Novice Ruth for letting me into their home and their lives, and showing me their great hospitality and love.

Helen Batten

CONTENTS

CHAPTER ONE
THE CALL

My first memory is the sound of an air-raid warning; I can only have been three. I was playing outside in the streets when a ghostly wail filled my head. I put my hands over my ears and ran in to my mother. I was crying 'stop it, Mummy, stop the noise', but she just grabbed my arm and pulled me under the kitchen table. Growing up in North London during the war, we were to spend a lot of time under the kitchen table and even more time in the dark, damp, communal air-raid shelter that our council block shared. But my father refused to let us be evacuated. For him, the war brought back too many difficult memories, and he kept his children close.

Probably the most important moment in our family's history was when father rode a war horse into the German guns at the beginning of the First World War. He didn't come from a privileged background, but he was tall and dashing and very good with horses. I was slightly puzzled as to how he had managed to become such a horse expert, growing up in poverty in Camden Town, unless he had spent time nuzzling up to the working horses that were still plodding up and down the streets.

He was the eldest of six children (six others having died) and my grandpa was a bounder. But my grandmother kept her children fed and clothed by taking in laundry. This tireless lady not only took care of their physical needs but also, perhaps inspired by the trauma of living with such an errant husband, paid great attention to their moral foundations. The motto drummed into them was 'Good, better, best. Never let it rest until the good is better and the better is best', with the result that as soon as war was declared Dad lied about his age and found himself at the age of 17 charging the Germans across the fields of Belgium.

It was only a few months before he was brought off his horse. We'd beg Mother to show us the wallet that had been in his breast pocket. It had a smoky hole right through the leather where the shrapnel had shot through his breastplate, and lodged in his lungs. We'd gaze in awe at the evidence of the event – the canvas upon which our whole family life was painted.

One day my sister asked Father what was the most physically painful thing he had ever experienced. We listened spellbound as he told us how the army medics had packed the wounds in his chest and arm with gauze soaked with salt, then left him for three days lying in this no-man's-land as the battle raged around him. Father had nothing to help relieve his pain, only Kipling's poem 'If' to fortify him (my grandmother's favourite),

And so hold on when there is nothing in you, except the Will which says to them: "Hold on!

He described the moment when they were finally able to come back and take him to hospital and unpack his wounds, taking out the gauze which had putrefied in the dirt and heat. But the moment his voice wavered was when he told us how they shot his wounded horse – the horse that Father believed had saved his life. At times I have felt as if I have been posted to the front line of human suffering; but one of the things that never ceases to amaze me is the resilience of the human spirit. I suppose Father was my first example.

When he arrived back in England, Father was sent to a special hospital in East London and my grandmother went to visit him. She'd never been to this area of London before and it was quite difficult for her to find the money for the fare. When she eventually walked into the ward she thought there had been a mistake. Father's face was covered in bandages, so still, and so at peace that she thought she'd come all this way only to find him dead. She went over to his bedside, took his cold hand and started to pray. My grandmother had already lost six of her 12 children and she wasn't prepared to part with this boy who was so brave and of whom she was so proud. He was her eldest. After a few minutes, the 'corpse' opened his eyes and smiled at her. From that moment Father thrived. He had lost the use of his right arm (he always wore a black leather glove and one of our jobs every morning was to do up his cufflinks), and he suffered debilitating bouts of bronchitis from the shrapnel left in his lungs, but he recovered his good looks and his optimism and within a couple of years he was married and working for the Post Office.

Father's war experience had a profound impact on us children in all sorts of ways, not least because he came out of hospital a fervent Socialist. Influenced by some of the soldiers he had met while he was recovering, the conclusion he had come to from the suffering of the war was that power had to be taken out of the hands of the elite and given to those who would actually have to fight. His first action when he left hospital was to walk into the local Labour Party office and sign up. I remember sitting at my father's feet listening to him talk about the evils of inequality, 'Is it right that some people have too much, while some people have too little, Katie? It's up to you and me and all of us to do something about it and we must keep on striving until this is put right.'

Of course this meant that Father had little time for religion – an establishment conspiracy to keep the workers in their place. We never went to church, but when I trotted down the road to see my grandmother, with a wink she would get out the family Bible and entrance me with stories of floods and arks, multi-coloured dreamcoats, wicked women cutting off their strong husband's hair, and virgin births in stables. It was our little secret. Meanwhile Father was working very hard, educating us in his own way.

One of the wonders of being the Second World War generation growing up in London was that if you had enlightened parents, it was possible to have a fantastically enriching, full education and Father was dedicated to instructing us – I was intimately acquainted with many museums, and frequently taken to watch Shakespeare at the Old Vic. Of course we had to sit up in the gods, but still, in a drab post-war London without television, that left quite an impression. I even remember Father taking me to see cricket at Lord's.

My mother was quietly complicit in all this socialism and self-improvement. She taught us to read at an early age and we grew up with a strong sense of right and wrong. She was a great household manager – highly organised and efficient, with complete knowledge and control of her household. She managed to work the household finances so that although we were poor, we didn't feel it. There was always spare food so that when friends and family popped round she was able to set another place at the table. Father worked as hard as his fragile health allowed, but when he was laid up in bed with one of his frequent bouts of bronchitis, Mother took in sewing.

My mother's controlled competence made the story of the way she fell in love with Father all the more puzzling. It seemed rather unlikely. Mother was not my father's first wife. Very soon after he left hospital, Father had fallen deeply in love with another woman and they had married and quickly had three children. Then, during one of my father's periods in hospital with chest complaints, his first wife had suddenly died, from consumption. Father was so ill he wasn't allowed to go to her funeral, but they rerouted the procession so it went past the house. The story goes that he said his last goodbye to her as her horse-driven hearse moved slowly past his window.

Father actually met my mother on his next stay in hospital. She happened to be a trainee nurse working on his ward. She was much younger than he, she was 24 years old, while my father was 38. Apparently it was love at first sight, which I suppose was not totally surprising because, despite his appalling health, Father still looked like Clark Gable. They did make a tall, striking couple. However, their families were not impressed by their relationship, so Mother and Father agreed to test their love by not seeing each other for six months. They lasted two weeks. Within the year Mother had given up work and was looking after my half-brother and sisters and I was on the way. Four years later my little brother, Harry, was born. Despite there being 16 years between my eldest half-sister, Elsie, and I, the two families always felt like one. We were a happy, secure family unit. My mother was particularly undemonstrative (even withering, sometimes) but somehow I did know that I was loved.

But the heart of the family was my father. So when he became really ill in the spring of 1948, we were all quietly scared. He took to his bed as the weather warmed up and I knew something was different: something about the way he was breathing, the way he was coughing. One day Mother took me aside and said, 'You know, Katie, Father might not get better.' I nodded, a horrible lump in my throat. I knew already, I could smell it in the air of the house. I would stand in the sitting room directly below their bedroom and listen. I counted the gaps between his heavy painful breaths, trying to work out if he was getting better or worse. I was ten; old enough not to be able to ask anyone what was going on. One afternoon, I was in the living room, listening. It all went quiet. I was trying to work out if this was a good or a bad sign when Mother came downstairs and said, 'Katie, Father has died.' My first thought was 'How on earth are we going to survive?' It seemed impossible that the family could carry on and not fall apart without him.

Of course we did survive. My big brother started giving Mum his wages and my smart eldest sister (who otherwise would probably have gone to university) left school and became a secretary to help support the family. But I struggled with the Father-shaped gap that had been left behind and all the unanswered questions that were left in his place. Principally, 'where have you gone?'

One sunny afternoon in the spring, six months after my father's death, I walked past our parish church and then I turned right round and walked in. Totally spontaneously, for the first time in my life, I found myself in a church. Suddenly, it seemed that here was a place where I might find the answer to my question. I sat in the pew in the dark and I felt comfortable and peaceful, at home in a way that I hadn't felt at home in our flat since Father had died. So the next Sunday I slipped out and went to morning communion and before I knew it, I was going to church every week. I didn't tell anyone because I knew it wouldn't go down well.

Of course it wasn't long before my secret was rumbled. One Sunday morning my big sister, Elsie, saw me coming out from the morning service and went straight home to Mother. 'I know where Katie's been going, Mum. Church.'

Mother raised an eyebrow. I kept very still.

'I caught her coming out of St Luke's this morning.'

Mother looked at me over the top of her glasses, 'I'm sure it's just a phase, isn't it, Katie?'

I didn't say anything. I knew it wasn't just a 'phase'. I also knew my mother well enough not to confront her.

Before long I was singing in the choir and making friends in the youth club, then I was confirmed. No one stopped me, although Mother made passing remarks about my 'religious mania' and although no one except my grandmother approved of religion, their disapproval was outweighed by their belief in personal freedom, so I was allowed to go about my spiritual business. Also, they were all struggling with their own grief and I think they thought it was my way of getting through and I'd grow out of it. The thing is, I didn't.

Unlike my clever brothers and sisters, I was really rather hopeless at school. I remember overhearing two of the primary school teachers who had taught my big sisters saying to each other, right in front of me, 'Oh, I don't know what's happened to Katie! Her sisters were always so bright.'

'Yes, strange isn't it? From the same family and yet so different.'

School just didn't inspire me. Again, unlike my gregarious siblings, I was quite shy and I stuttered when I had to read aloud in class. Most of the time I was caught up in a world of my own: I collected stamps and knitted big woolly jumpers and I was terribly disorganised. I was always wearing games kit on the wrong days and forgetting my homework. It's not that I wasn't interested in learning – I read everything I could get my hands on and I loved going to see plays – but I was only interested if it was my own choice and school was not my own choice. So unlike my siblings I finished primary school at the bottom of the class and failed my 11-plus. To the shame of the family I was the only Crisp not to go to grammar school and I had to shuffle down to the local secondary modern instead. I guess I was quite headstrong in my own quiet way. Church was my choice and my thing, my own little separate existence if you like, and, greatly to my own surprise, I began to make a bit of a mark. I started to help organise the youth club, then I was running it and suddenly I found myself in charge of the youth conference for the diocese of London. It seems I had a secret abilities. Again 'religious mania' was all my mother would say on the subject.

When I reached 16, I left school with absolutely no qualifications. There was a family conference around the kitchen table. My big brother and sisters were there. Even my grandmother had been summoned.

'So, Katie, what do you want to do?' Mother asked.

'I'd like to be an actress.'

There was a stunned silence.

'Shall I ask you that question again, Katie?' Mother said slowly. 'Now please tell us what you have in mind to do now you have left school.'

I was feeling less confident now. 'No really, Mother. I'd like to be an actress. I know it might seem strange but I'm not shy when I'm on stage. Really! Miss Woodridge thinks I've got real talent.'

I could see big sister Elsie trying not to laugh. Edward was staring very hard at the table. I soldiered on, 'You know how much I've always enjoyed going to the theatre ...' (actually I saw myself as more of a blonde Vivien Leigh, but I knew any mention of *Gone with the Wind* would finish them off).

But my grandmother had already had enough.

'What rubbish, Katie, I can't believe I'm hearing this! I thought you had more sense. Acting! Tshhhh,' she shook her head. 'Well, I've heard it all now. You've spent too much time at the pictures and not enough at your homework. Look, my girl, you've got to earn a living. Acting is not a living. If you want to eat, you've got to work.'

And that was the end of that. I got a job working in a surveyor's office and I was sent off to night school to try and pass the exams I should have passed at school. I absolutely hated it. Shorthand, it drove me insane. Or at least it would have driven me insane if I hadn't been hatching a plan.

One of the turning points in my life was the day the Americans dropped a bomb on Hiroshima. Father had sent me down to the corner shop to get his paper. On the cover was the most horrific photograph I had ever seen. They really did show photographs of the terrible injuries from the atom bomb. There were lots of them inside. I couldn't believe that the Americans and, as their allies, we, had done this to other human beings. Then nine days later they did it all over again at Nagasaki. A feeling of disgust stayed with me and it got me thinking. As I got older I started to dream about travelling so I could get to know people in other corners of the world, perhaps people who didn't look like us, who were poorer and needed help. I wanted to do something meaningful and useful, to do something my father would have been proud of. There was one obvious way I could do this and that was to become a missionary, not the preaching kind of missionary, but perhaps one of the teaching or nursing kinds. Becoming a missionary was not as radical an option as it would be today. Think of it as more like taking a gap year. Missionary work was one of the few respectable routes for a working class and unqualified woman to travel and see the world. In 1954 it was perfectly acceptable to live away from home and mix with other young people (including men) if you were being chaperoned by the Church of England.

I started training at the Society for the Propagation of the Gospel. The problem was you had to go where you were sent and they wanted to send me off to India for five years. Suddenly I wasn't sure, the one thing I knew was it would kill my mother. I stalled. Then one day I went to the wedding of one of my church friends. Drifting round the reception in a rather smart outfit I felt a hand on my arm. I looked round. It belonged to a handsome young curate.

'I say, I do like your hat. Will you come and work for me?' he said.

I blushed. He was rather extraordinary, but I liked the cut of his gib. 'It depends what kind of work you are offering,' I replied.

'Something that will change your life,' he said.

I needed no more encouragement. When my theological education was complete, I started a new job as a parish worker for All Saints Church in Poplar.

However this wasn't a case of 'living happily ever after'. In fact it was a long time before I felt happy at all. On my first evening in the parish I put my suitcase on my bed and burst into tears.

Poplar was full of docks, and I was surrounded by a level of poverty that I had never seen before. Until I had got used to it, it was quite intimidating, even for a working-class girl from Camden Town. It was also hard, hard work. The parish of All Saints was huge. We were expected to get up early and work very late. Saturday was our day off, but we still had to stay up late to clean up the church hall after whichever wedding reception or dance had hired it, and get the hall ready for church activities the next day.

My main job was visiting the parishioners and helping to run the South Poplar Youth Club (or Spy). It ran six nights a week and had over 300 members. In some ways this was fantastic, we were an important presence in a really deprived area and we were doing a lot of good work in the community. But my heart ached for some of the tatty children – they were dirty and sometimes shoeless. In Camden Town, everyone had shoes, even during the war.

Tenements like Canada Buildings were awful. You went in them and there would be little furniture, but plenty of unwelcome wildlife; insects I'd never known existed. They made our council flat look like a palace. I didn't understand why sometimes these homes were quite so unclean. There were a lot of unconventional happenings among the community. I'd never even heard of incest before I arrived in Poplar. It was an education, really.

But as I got used to the conditions, I began to see that beneath the grime and poverty, the people were extraordinary. They were a tight-knit community that generally looked after each other, a closer community in fact than we'd had in Camden Town. The people were warm, friendly and funny. If they accepted you, which generally they did, they would do anything for you. Of course it was fun too. We were a crowd of young people working together, all from different backgrounds and different parts of the country. That was also part of the education. The handsome young curate was right – my new job was starting to change my life.

One of my weekly duties was to go round the parish with the Reverend Granger, helping him to give Communion to those parishioners who could no longer make it to church. It was a cheery late spring afternoon when we set off to see Old Sue. Everyone greeted us as we walked along – working men tugged their caps, women in their overalls called out 'Hello, Father' from their doorsteps and shoeless children trotted behind us. Despite the bombed-out ruins, the stray dogs and the litter strewn across the pavement, it was difficult not to feel happy. I was beginning to sense the value of feeling welcomed, accepted and maybe even respected in this friendly community. Since being at All Saints I had pondered my father's belief that some people had too little and some people had too much. Too much or too little of what? He was talking about money, but I was no longer sure that was all that mattered.

Old Sue was a well-known East End 'character'. Rounder than she was tall and always saying something forthright, she lived in one of the old tenement buildings. She didn't have much of a life – she couldn't get out and was effectively trapped in her flat. It was a pretty squalid flat too, never cleaned and with a lavatory right in the kitchen. I had a morbid fascination with this toilet. Old Sue was lucky to have one at all – many people had to share the communal lavatories on the ground floor. But still, a toilet stuck randomly in the middle of the kitchen? I wondered about privacy and food preparation, but Old Sue was far too fierce to ask and I thought the Reverend might not appreciate my curiosity.

With the benefit of experience I had come prepared with a packet of mints. There were certain people's homes that smelled so foul I could only enter with a mint between my teeth, otherwise I might be sick. Old Sue's was one of those places.

As the Reverend knocked on the door I popped a pepper-mint puff in my mouth. No answer. I was thinking 'Hurry up, Old Girl, or I'll have to use up another mint'. The Reverend knocked again; still no answer. He was starting to look worried.

'Katie, go and grab that bobby over there and see if he can help us force this door. I don't like the look of this.'

So I ran down the stairs after the policeman. He was only too pleased to help and it didn't take much of a shove to force the front door open. There was Old Sue lying on the floor, struggling. As we knelt down beside her we could see one side of her face had collapsed. She was trying to speak but her face was so twisted we couldn't make out the words. Reverend Granger didn't waste any time. 'Go and get one of the Sisters, quick,' he said.

All Saints Church was on one side of a large Georgian square in Poplar. On the other side of the square was an old Mission House, where five or so nuns and a handful of nurses lived. I really didn't know much about these women, except that for the last 100 years this Anglican order of nursing sisters, the Community of St John the Divine, had been caring for the local people from cradle to grave. I had watched them coming and going on their bikes, heavily laden with medical equipment, but I had never felt the urge to introduce myself. I was slightly repelled by the Sisters' blue habits and all they represented. Only the month before I had been sitting on a train when a nun came and sat down opposite me. 'Oh crikey! I hope that never happens to me,' I thought. She looked perfectly content, but I felt slightly anxious sitting next to her, like if I got too close I might catch her vocation.

Now I had no choice but to come face-to-face with them. I ran down the streets and for the first time, pulled the bell on the heavy door of the house. It seemed all locked up and quiet. I pulled the bell again. Then I heard slow, echoing steps getting closer. There was a jangling of locks and the door slowly opened. In front of me was an old nun, with the palest of skin. My eyes were drawn to the enormous silver cross hanging round her neck. It seemed like a declaration of total confident faith. I also noticed the gold ring on the third finger of her right hand, a sign of her consecration to Christ. This was Sister Dorothy.

'Good afternoon, Sister, I'm sorry to disturb you but Reverend Granger has asked me to come and get you. It's Old Sue. We found her collapsed in her flat. I think she's had a stroke.'

Sister Dorothy peered over the top of her glasses with what, if she hadn't been in Holy Orders, I might have taken to be a look of disdain. 'Oh, diagnosis as well,' she said. 'Well, I'll get my bag and you'd better take me down there, hadn't you?'

We walked along in silence. I felt too intimidated to speak and Sister Dorothy obviously didn't feel the need to. When we got there, she pronounced that Old Sue had indeed had a stroke and sent the Reverend off to fetch an ambulance.

'All right, young lady,' she said, 'you had better help me get these clothes off.' I was slightly dismayed. I really didn't want to touch Old Sue. She was wearing lots of layers that didn't appear to have been removed for months and the smell was overpowering. But as I slowly and gently helped to undress this sick old lady, my revulsion evaporated and I was filled with a sense of compassion that I'd never experienced before. It was then that I had my vision.

I saw myself dressed as a nun. I was wearing a blue habit with a white veil covering my long hair and there was a heavy silver cross hanging from my neck.

'No, no, no,' screamed the voice in my head. 'I like nail varnish too much!'

But even as I had the thought, Sister Dorothy turned around and looked at me, and said, 'Well, what are you going to do about it then?'

'About what?'

'Well, I think we both know, don't we?'

I'd never wanted to become a nun. It seemed like such an extraordinary loss of freedom; something I could never see myself doing. I was young. I wanted to do what I wanted, when I wanted; and anyway, I liked nail varnish and everything it stood for – clothes, parties, and yes, men – far, far too much …

But then I had just seen myself, with my own eyes, and Sister Dorothy had obviously seen it too. It sent a cold feeling of dread to the pit of my stomach. But when I got back to the parish house and heard that Old Sue had died, I was filled with a sense of gratitude that I had been able to help her in her last hours. The act of making her feel comfortable as she passed from this world felt like a privilege and my faith felt stronger, as if I had just taken just a small step closer to the Divine.

But not that much closer to the Divine. The next day I had my regular weekly meeting with my spiritual director, Father David. These meetings were supposed to be a discussion about my progress as a parish worker. Instead he opened the conversation with a surprise question, 'So, Katie, have you considered becoming a nun?'

I felt cornered. I hadn't said anything to him. How did he know? I felt as if there was a heavenly conspiracy going on and I didn't like it. 'I don't think so. I don't think I'm the right material at all,' I said.

He raised his eyebrows at me. 'Are you sure? Do you even know what the right material is? Might there be something to be gained by a little further investigation. Just to make sure …?'

I sensed a challenge. 'Oh, all right then. I'll give it a little further investigation – if only to prove I'm utterly unsuitable.'

Father David smiled enigmatically.

In the absence of knowing any other nuns, I found myself writing to Mother Sarah Grace, the Mother Superior of our neighbours in the Mission House.

The Community of St John the Divine was set up with the express purpose of nursing the poor. It's hard to believe now, but back in the early Victorian age the reputation of nurses was quite unsavoury – think of Dickens's 'Mrs Gamp' and picture a low-class woman of dubious character, dirty and drunk. This was the public profile of the early nineteenth-century nurse. They were seen as grasping and thieving; there were even reports of nurses offering immoral services late at night in the male wards for financial reward. So it certainly wasn't the kind of profession that would either attract or be permitted for respectable ladies. When Robert Bentley Todd was appointed a professor of King's College medical school, he came to the conclusion that despite the new innovations in medicine, his patients were still dying because of the appalling standards of these nurses, not least their lack of hygiene. Very much a man of his time, Todd believed that professionalism at work came from a person having a strong religious and moral underpinning. The Victorians loved the saying 'Cleanliness is next to Godliness'. So Todd decided that if he could only impose the moral discipline of the religious life on his nurses, their work would be transformed.

In 1848 Todd summoned a meeting of great and good gentlemen (including some of the bishops of the Church of England) to discuss forming a religious community in which women would receive not only clinical training, but also be educated in his words, 'to regard their work as a religious one affording special opportunities for the exercise of Christian love and womanly tenderness'. He wanted to develop a class of nurses who would regard their work as a religious calling. At this time the Roman Catholic Church still inspired enormous fear and suspicion throughout the population, so Todd and his colleagues were determined to ensure the Sisters of St John looked very different to Catholic nuns. It was decided that there would be 'no vows, no poverty, no monastic obedience, no celibacy, no engagements, no cloistered seclusion, no tyranny exercised over will or conscience; but a full, free and willing devotion to the cause of Christian charity'.

Also, in keeping with the rigid class divisions of the time, it was decided that the Sisters could only come from the upper echelons of society. To ensure this, the Sisters were not only unpaid but had to give £50 a year (the equivalent of around £3,000 today) to the Community. They would live in a house under the supervision of a master and lady superintendent and were to train working-class women to be paid assistant nurses.

The new Community was surprisingly radical for its day. It actually offered the first opportunity for an upper-class woman to have a full-time working career without losing her status as a lady. To me, in 1958, becoming a nun seemed like a big sacrifice of personal freedom, but for a mid-Victorian lady it was the only opportunity to legitimately escape getting married and the dangerous business of having endless numbers of children. Instead it allowed women to lead an independent life, do constructive work and live in a comfortable home where they could make their own rules. It also offered the working-class nurses they employed one of the few routes to improve their social status. This meant that from the start, the Community of St John tended to attract rather pioneering, wilful women – women who today we might call feminists. Perhaps I was more suited to the Community than I first realised.

However, the Sisters of St John were first and foremost nurses, so when I wrote to the Mother Superior expressing an interest in knowing more about her Community, I was pretty confident that she would tell me to go away and come back if and when I had managed to become a nurse. But this is the letter I got back:

Dear Miss Crisp,

Thank you for your enquiry regarding the Community of St John the Divine. I am delighted that you would like to get to know us better with a view to testing your vocation to the religious life.

You are quite right that in the past it has only been possible to accept into the novitiate ladies who have already been awarded their General Nurse's Certificate. However at our Chapter meeting this week we voted to change this rule, and from now on it will be possible for ladies to both train to be nuns and train to be nurses at the same time. Perhaps this is an example of Divine Providence? It certainly seems that God is smoothing your path to us. With this in mind I would like to invite you to come and join us, initially for a year. Unless I hear otherwise, we will expect to see you at the Mother House in Hastings, on January 25th. In the meantime we will pray for you.

May God bless you,
Mother Sarah Grace

I was slightly wrong-footed by this letter and the phrase went through my head 'you can run, but you can't hide'. I was a bit shocked but it did seem as if this really was my calling. But I still had to face one last obstacle: my family.

I took a day off especially to go and see them. I was dreading it, but tempting as it might be, I couldn't see how I could go to Hastings and enter the novitiate without actually telling them. Running away to become a nun didn't seem to be starting off on the right foot.

However, Mother just said, 'Well, that's not news. I'm just surprised it took you so long.' That was it.

My siblings were more difficult. 'How ridiculous!' Edward snorted. I knew he was actually embarrassed by me. But it was my biggest sister Elsie's reaction that was most upsetting. By this time she was married and had settled down happily with her husband and two children. She put her head on the kitchen table and sobbed.

'Oh, Katie, please don't! Everything you will give up. Such a waste. Please think again.'

'I can't help it. I really can't – I don't have a choice. I know this is difficult for you to understand but I believe God has called me.'

'Oh, stop it! I won't hear it. I think you are going mad, Katie. Mother should have taken you to the doctor or something years ago. Please don't do it.'

It was horrible, but it was done and nobody ever said anything again. They didn't need to. I knew they disapproved, but I also knew that they still loved me. The way was now open for me to travel to Hastings and to the Mother House.

There's a popular misconception that a nun becomes a nun because that's something she's always wanted to do. Perhaps when you see a nun you see someone who was not brave enough for the world, someone who wanted to escape. But usually it's quite the opposite. A nun, before she became a nun, probably had the same kind of hopes and dreams for her future as you do. She probably didn't want to escape the world but rather to escape from God. But over the years I've seen it happen many times – when God calls, you can run and run, but He'll always catch you in the end.

This is the way that He caught me.

CHAPTER TWO
BUT WHY?

From the very beginning I was the square peg of a feisty girl facing a bit of a round hole. I look back now and I'm reminded of when you get a new pair of shoes and they need to be worn in before the blisters stop. But is it the shoe that adjusts to the shape of the foot, or the foot that has to adjust to the shape of the shoe? The problem was that in 1958 the Community didn't bend for anyone, so if I was to stay, it was me that was going to have to fundamentally change shape.

'But why?' – the question that kept going through my head and coming out of my mouth all through that first year at the convent. There was so much that didn't make sense, that seemed ridiculous, that was turning me from a grown woman into a child. Within days of arriving I felt like a naughty schoolgirl seeking out opportunities to subvert the system: I had arrived in a sausage factory turning out perfectly moulded, cloned nuns, and I was damned if they were going to do that to me. I had a real feeling that my self had to be preserved at all costs, even if it was disguised under a veil and sensible knickers.

Ah yes, the knickers. Before I had even got there, all my worries were confirmed when they sent me a list of what I had to bring. It included

- *Knickers: white with legs*
- *Vests*
- *Full-length navy blue dressing gown*
- *Full-length nightgown with buttons to the neck and long sleeves.*

You will be provided with three postulant's dresses once you arrive, so there is no need to bring any other clothing, except to avoid waste you may bring your old night attire to use until it wears out.

You may also bring three books of a suitable nature.

Which sort of summed up the whole of my first year, which turned out to be a clash between the bizarre and the mundane with the seriously, profoundly spiritual.

Knickers with legs? I had no idea what they might be and even less idea where I might find them, so I decided to take the risk that nobody was going to check and packed my current lacey things. I eventually tracked down a long, sensible Victorian nightgown in Peter Jones department store. For a few minutes I was too embarrassed to ask for one. 'Jesus, give me courage,' I prayed and then I told the shop assistant, 'It's for my grandmother.'

The books were much easier. I took a book of prayers that my godmother had given me when I was confirmed called *Daily Light*. It has a simple reading for each day of the year and I have used it frequently since. I often marvel at how much the meaning of a reading has changed when I get back to it a year later, which just goes to show we are perpetually changing even if it doesn't feel like it. I also took a book of spiritual poetry and *The Cloud of Unknowing*, a medieval mystical work offering guidance on how to reach God through letting go of the world and opening oneself up to whatever may occur. I guess I sensed I was about to embark on a risky spiritual journey.

So, despite all my reservations, I was making all the necessary preparations to leave, but still something deep inside of me must have seriously not wanted to go. On the night of one of the parish Christmas parties, I tripped on the freshly polished stairs, fell down two storeys and broke my ankle. As I sat in the hospital casualty department a host of conflicting thoughts went through my head. I had a lump in my throat because I had just ruined what might be my last chance to wear a pretty dress, have a drink, perhaps even have an innocent chat with a nice young man. But even as I fought back the tears, I realised that this accident might actually offer up the opportunity for more parties. I knew that I couldn't go to the convent in plaster, and I also knew that the Community would not take any new recruits during Lent, which usually starts at the end of February. This would give me until the beginning of the summer to remain at large in the outside world: a stay of execution, if you like. Even as I sat there in agony, I felt a wave of relief.

The relief only lasted until the first week in January, when this letter landed on the breakfast table.

Dear Miss Crisp,

We were all very sorry to hear about your accident. We hope and pray that your ankle is healing. It is a shame that you have had to postpone your arrival. However it is good news that your plaster will be removed at the beginning of March. As you know we cannot accept new postulants during Lent, but because Easter is late this year, Lent starts late. So we would like to invite you to start with us on Ash Wednesday, March 10th.

We will be praying for you in the meantime.

God's blessings be with you,
Mother Sarah Grace

So there was to be no stay of execution, and – more sinisterly – I was being summoned to enter the religious life on Ash Wednesday. Ash Wednesday is the day that marks the beginning of Lent and 40 days of fasting and abstinence. It is traditionally a day of repentance and the day when a cross of ash is put on the foreheads of the faithful to remind us that, just as we come from dust, we will return to dust. It seemed like a brutal reminder of the seriousness of the step I was about to take, not to mention the end of any party plans.

So at the beginning of March 1958 I packed my small bag with long nighties and vests. I gave away my more frivolous books to my niece, divided my nail varnish between my sisters, and gave my clothes to my girlfriends. I did, however, hold back my favourite party dress: a wool suit and a cashmere twinset. I secretly hid them at the back of a wardrobe in my mother's house as an insurance policy, just in case I didn't make it. My Plan B.

Meanwhile, my local bishop had a rather intuitive wife. A couple of weeks before I was due to leave she rang me.

'Hello, Katie, how are you? How's your ankle?'

'Oh, not bad, not bad at all. Plaster's off and I'm nearly walking normally.'

'Oh, I'm so glad to hear that. And I also hear that you will be off to the Community soon?'

'Yes. Yes, it seems that they can admit me on Ash Wednesday.'

'Well, that's what I'd heard. Look, I've been thinking: the Bishop and I would like to invite you over for lunch, a sort of celebration if you like, on your day of departure and then we could take you to the station and put you on the train. Save your family having to do it. Give you a really good send-off.'

I paused to think it through. I had a feeling she was really saying, 'Save you and your family the distress of seeing you off'. I appreciated her kindness and accepted her invitation. So, on the day of my departure I went to lunch with the Bishop and his wife and then they both took me to the train and cheerily waved me off. What might have been an agonising moment is now a happy memory.

Two hours later I found myself on the platform of Hastings station with an elderly nun in a blue habit slowly working her way towards me with her arms outstretched.

'Hello, dear, you must be Katie. Welcome.'

She placed her hands on my shoulders and studied me. I felt embarrassed by the intensity of her gaze and her long silence, as if she could see straight to my doubts and shallowness, and the thoughts of nail varnish and parties. It took some effort not to look away. Then the spell was broken.

'I'm Sister Clemence. I'm very lucky, you know. There are only two of us who can drive, which means I get to do the station run and get out.'

I thought I detected a twinkle in her eye.

In the car park was an old yellow Morris Minor. It was going green at the edges and had a 'Jesus Lives' sticker in the back window. Sister Clemence struggled into the driving seat. She turned the ignition and the car proceeded to lurch forward with a horrible grating sound – 'Whoops! The handbrake. Silly me!'

She released the brake and the car shot forward and bumped into the parked car in front. Sister Clemence didn't seem the slightest bit concerned. We advanced to the Mother House at 30 miles per hour, lurching in second gear into the centre of the road, with cars scattering to avoid us. Sister Clemence chatted away to me, oblivious to the hooting drivers and shocked pedestrians.

'So dear, we have 16 sisters, four novices and, let me think,' she swerved and hit the kerb, 'just one other postulant, Cecilia, in the house.'

I wasn't worried by Sister Clemence's driving – her complete serenity was infectious. I wondered whether this was what a lifetime of working on your faith brought you. I was also trying hard not to laugh.

'Here we go. Welcome to the Mother House.'

Up a long drive banked by rhododendrons was a large Victorian house. It had big windows, turrets and wings, but it was not imposing. Perhaps it was the large windows making me think of kindly eyes looking out on the world or the borders creating a welcome path. It was surrounded by lawns, with protective woodland encircling them, and looked like a comfortable Victorian country estate, which men in plus-fours and ladies with parasols might appear from at any moment. I was filled with emotion.

The Mother House is the name given to the headquarters of a Community of Sisters, because it's a family home. When you enter a Community you give up your own home and enter a new home and family, probably forever. A home is a place where you go out from and return to, a place of safety. Home should be a place where you can be yourself. Could I be myself here? It was a long way from where I had grown up in Camden Town. I had been worried that the Mother House might look like a prison, but it didn't. This house was drawing me up and into its arms.

'Please God, can it be a home and not a prison,' I prayed.

Sister Clemence interrupted my reverie. 'So what do you think of your new home, Katie?'

'I feel a bit like Dorothy in *The Wizard of Oz*, when she comes out of the forest and sees the Emerald City for the first time.'

'Oh goodness, I hope we can live up to your expectations. You are a poet!' she exclaimed.

As the car crashed over another bump and swerved to avoid the rhododendrons, she chuckled, 'It's a pity Dorothy didn't have a Morris Minor – it might have saved her a whole lot of trouble.'

I wasn't so sure.

When we arrived I was taken straight to see the Mother Superior, Sarah Grace. I walked down the corridor behind Sister Clemence with not a little trepidation. Like my first encounter with the Mother House, this first meeting with the Mother Superior seemed very important. Would

I like her, and would she like me? Could we do business together?

It's no accident that the head of a female religious community is usually called the Mother Superior. She is elected by the Community to have authority over them. She is expected to show strong leadership, to be the chief interpreter of the monastic rules and a prophet of God's will for the Community. She is supposed to be a mother to you, who guides and protects you; but also to be obeyed in all things. She sets the boundaries. There's something of a test of faith at the heart of your relationship with the Mother Superior, faith that, even when it might not seem like it, she has your best interests at heart. I had to ask her permission for everything I now wanted to do. And with no money, anything I wanted or needed, even down to the smallest tube of toothpaste, I had to write and ask for. I'd had more freedom when I was ten years old.

This maternal role was set out very clearly by the founding fathers of the Community. In their original mission statement they stipulated that the Mother Superior had to be over 35 years of age and a member of the Church of England with a baptismal record to prove it. She also had to be able 'to conduct all things to the honour and glory of God, showing kindness without weakness, firmness without severity, and act in all things with sincerity, truth and love, in a spirit of self-denial and resignation to the Divine will'.

However, just as in those times a family was seen to be incomplete without a strong father at the helm, the Community was to have a Master. Not only was he to take the three services a day, but constantly interview the nurses and sisters privately at the end of each day, keeping in mind their individual weaknesses, questioning them as to their conduct to make sure it was done with holy reverence. It was made very clear that he had ultimate authority over the Mother Superior.

The first Mother Superior they found, or rather who found them, was Mary Jones. She arrived on the convent doorstep one day offering to be a paid housekeeper. At first the governing council refused. It was a principle of the sisterhood that 'the Sisters set an example of Christian humility for the working-class women by working without pay'. Within a week the council had relented and given Mary Jones a salary of £20 and within a year she had been appointed to be in charge with the Chaplain. She wrote,

'I am most fully resolved, for our safety and our credit and our comfort, to have the rules literally obeyed, and that too, willingly and cheerfully. Anything in the shape of disobedience or insubordination shall be instantly repressed.'

So Mary Jones was strict with her nurses, but, like a good mother, she was also hawkish in protecting them. She believed that seven hours' sleep was not enough for the night nurses and insisted they should have eight. She also asked that the night nurses be allowed a candle on night duty as well as the low gas light and she encouraged them to knit.

'It is dreary work indeed to watch in a large ward with only the glimmering of the gas turned down very low,' she said.

Sister Mary Jones was somewhat legendary in the Community. The Bishop's wife had looked out a photo of her for me – all stiff white bonnet, stern face and buttoned-down bosom. She had been best friends with Florence Nightingale and they used to go on holiday together. Indeed in a letter to Florence Nightingale, Sister Mary Jones said that a Mother Superior should have a 'mother's feeling for, and sympathy with, her nurses'. She should be 'a large-hearted, loving Christian woman, clear-sighted and firm – but forbearing and patient'. I wondered how Mother Sarah Grace would measure up.

The Reverend Mother's study was small and sparse. The only furniture was a bureau and a desk, and there were no photos or pictures on the wall, only a simple crucifix. The room was dominated by the large window with its view across the lawns to the forest beyond. Mother Sarah Grace was a small, fragile-looking woman, with an aura of calm and that struck me as real holiness. Right from the start I was in awe of this tiny, serious person. Like Sister Clemence, she regarded me intently in a long moment of silence. I felt myself blushing once again. Was I supposed to speak? In the end she broke the silence.

'Welcome, Katie, we are so pleased to have you here at last. I hope you will find that the Mother House becomes a home for you.'

'Yes, Mother, I am glad to be here.'

I hoped I sounded like I meant it. I *thought* I meant it. Anyway, I was determined to give it my best shot. She continued.

'New members bring the potential for new life and talents to our community.' She paused; I didn't know whether I was supposed to speak. Was I supposed to offer an opinion of what talents I might bring? My mind went blank. All I could think of was my stamp collection. Luckily I held back this thought and she went on, 'Your time as a postulant will be the first test of your vocation. It will mean taking part in the life and duties of the sisterhood, so you and I can discover if you have the spirit and wisdom to set out on the path of holy growth.'

Path of holy growth? I began to feel scared.

'The road to life profession is a long journey. We need to discover if you are genuinely called to our way of life and have the basic qualities necessary. We will seek to find out if you have a love of Our Lord, a desire to pray, a call to ministry, and flexibility in all things.'

I thought those qualities might apply to me (although I wasn't entirely sure about the flexibility); but what about all my other 'qualities' that weren't mentioned? My humour, my temper, my scattiness – where might they fit into this new home?

'So, Katie, you have taken the first step on the very bottom rung of the long ladder that takes you towards becoming a Sister, your life vows, and a journey towards grace and deeper communion with the Almighty Father. This journey could take at the very least seven years, for some it takes longer and many never make it at all.'

She paused so I could take this in.

'Anyway, for now let's just concentrate on your first step. After six months of being a postulant, if it seems right, you will be offered the opportunity to take the next step, that is, to be accepted as a novice. I will be your Novice Mistress and guide you during these early days. Is everything clear?'

'Yes, Mother, I understand.'

What I understood from this was that I was about to be judged, and I could feel myself already getting rebellious.

'One last thing – you will no longer be known as Katie. From now on you will be called Catherine Mary.'

With that I was dismissed.

Sister Clemence was waiting outside to take me to my room. She looked at me quizzically.

'So, Katie, what am I to call you now?'

'Um … Catherine Mary, I think.'

She looked at me sympathetically.

'Well, Catherine Mary, I expect you're feeling a bit overwhelmed. Don't worry, we've all felt that way. You'll get used to it, it's about getting into the rhythm of the place. It will become your rhythm before you know it.'

'Really?'

'Oh yes. One day you'll wake up and realise it's all second nature.'

On that note, she cheerily opened the door to a room with two beds in it. It was small, but warm and cosy and I could again see it was dominated by the view of the forest stretching out across the horizon.

'You're sharing with our second newest recruit, Cecilia. She's working at the moment, but she'll be back soon. Unpack, my dear.'

She went to leave, then spun round.

'Oh yes, in the next day or so let me cut your hair. Don't delay, otherwise Mother Sarah Grace will do it and it will be a right old hatchet job. I promise you I'll cut it so that if you decide to leave, you can still walk in the outside world without a hat.'

I was horrified – my lovely, long, blonde hair! I'd thought I could just pin it back behind the veil. Before I could stop myself, I blurted out: 'But why?'

'Why, dear? Well, otherwise it's going to escape from your veil and then you'll get in no end of trouble and she'll just cut it off anyway. Best take matters in hand yourself. No room for vanity in this Community, I'm afraid.' Then she turned on her heel and left.

Finally on my own, I went over to the window and looked out. Trees as far as the eye could see. They were beautiful, an enchanted forest, but I had never lived anywhere where you couldn't see another house and plenty of people. I felt a pang for the bustle of my city. I actually missed the gas works. Again, I asked God to give me strength.

Luckily strength came in the form of my new roommate, Cecilia. She was willowy and elegant and spoke beautifully. I was quite taken aback. She walked into the bedroom we were to share and it was as if an angel in a postulant's dress had descended. She was just a few years older than me, but she had an aura of serenity way beyond her years.

'Hello. It's Catherine Mary, isn't it?'

'It seems I am.'

She laughed.

'I am so pleased to meet you and share a room with you. I have been praying for you to come for the last five months.'

'Gosh, no pressure then!'

Then we both laughed. I was taken aback by Cecilia's perfect elocution. She seemed so posh. Camden girl that I was, I couldn't help but feel intimidated by the thought that I was going to have to share with this lady who was so obviously 'top drawer'. In those days the class system was still very much in place and I really hadn't come into contact with many people from the upper class, certainly not in the kind of proximity that was demanded by sharing a room. One of the ways in which the Community was ahead of its time was bringing women of all backgrounds together and forming a community, a family, whatever our different backgrounds. I thought of something that St Benedict had written – that the bravest of monks was not the hermit, but the one who had learned to live with others in a Community. Perhaps the Mother House was not going to offer an escape from humanity but a lesson in how to deal with it. I remembered how the ancients of the Far East depicted hell as a place where people have chopsticks a yard long so they can't possibly feed themselves. In heaven the chopsticks are also a yard long, but the people feed each other. Was I capable of this?

However, sharing with Cecilia was not too difficult a test. She was especially careful to blend in, never alluding to her background except indirectly with her fox-hunting metaphors or when reading the paper she would casually say, 'Gosh, Johnny in a spot of bother again!' and you'd see she was talking about a member of the aristocracy. She immediately reached out to me by telling the story of her journey to the Mother House. Home from boarding school at the age of 15, she fell in love with a country vicar who had come to preach in her parish church. His sermon sent fire through her soul and for the first time she felt a spiritual connection to another human being. Unfortunately this other human being was married, but Cecilia was very determined and knew what she knew; that she'd found a soulmate of the religious kind.

Filled with passion, as soon as she got home, Cecilia wrote to the vicar telling him how she felt. She received a letter back by return of post. This was the start of a spiritual relationship where Cecilia and the vicar explored their feelings for God together. Cecilia knew there was no other man for her and she also knew that she could never have him in the worldly sense. She decided that there was no alternative but to dedicate herself to Christ and become a nun. Her family were horrified, her friends laughed, even her own parish priest (not the country vicar) told her to think again. She may have been stopped from going to a convent, but Cecilia absolutely refused to go out with any of the eligible young men who asked her out (Cecilia was beautiful, with long red hair) and instead further upset her parents by taking herself to secretarial college and getting a job.

One day she was called into the office of the owner, Mr Smith, who said, 'I like you a lot. I think you are a bright, hardworking, decent girl. I have to say, though, I have been watching you and I can't help noticing your heart really isn't in what you are doing.'

'Yes.'

'This job just isn't right for you, is it?'

'No. I'm sorry.'

'In that case – now this is really important – have you any idea what job would be right for you?'

'Oh yes, sir,' Cecilia smiled.

'Well, what is it then?'

'I want to become a nun.'

Incredibly, Mr Smith showed no sign of surprise. Instead he said, 'Then that is what you must become.'

For the first time (apart from the country vicar) Cecilia had found someone who took her seriously and she felt a huge relief. Mr Smith then went on to tell Cecilia how his eldest daughter had become a nun.

'She's found a peace and fulfilment in her life that few of us are ever lucky to find. Would you mind if I wrote to your father?'

So Mr Smith wrote to her father and one day Cecilia was called into her father's study and told that she had his blessing to go and join the Community. So Cecilia arrived at the Mother House and carried on her correspondence with the country vicar. They wrote letters to each other of a spiritual nature, where they shared their beliefs and the insights they were learning about the Divine. Cecilia only stopped writing on the day she was told of his death.

Cecilia guided me through those first tricky days. I was inspired by her calm obedience and yet I still had a panicky sense that I was losing something: a bit of my self was slipping through my fingers. I think the enforced strict hierarchy of the Community had something to do with it. For example, there was a rule that you had to curtsey to every Sister above you, and, as the most junior member of the Community, that meant I had to curtsey to everybody. At the end of the day my knees ached.

Mealtimes were solemn occasions. Except on feast days we had to eat in silence; the Mother Superior sat at the top of the long wooden table and dished up the food. The most junior member, again myself, had to take the plates along the rows of nuns, serving again according to seniority. This meant that if I didn't get a move on my food would be cold by the time I got to sit down. Not that the food was particularly exciting; it was basic and nourishing, but not always incredibly tasty. I'd been thrown in at the deep end by arriving at the start of Lent. The meals were particularly plain, with dry bread on Fridays for breakfast, and there was no break in the silence.

'Watch out for Sister Felicity,' Cecilia had warned. Sister Felicity? She was a very old Sister, partially deaf and blind, with a line of medicine bottles in front of her plate. I couldn't imagine what Cecilia was talking about. Then one day, just as I reached over the table and put the custard jug in front of her, I saw Sister Felicity pop her sleeping pills into the jug, looking at me all the while. She stared at me as if to say, 'Well, what are you going to do about it?' I stood rooted to the spot and watched as the jug went down the table, with the Sisters pouring laced custard over their apple crumble. I did nothing, but chuckled to myself and avoided the custard.

The next day I was summoned to the Mother Superior's office.

'Catherine Mary, it has come to my attention that you have been making complaints about the food.'

'Complaints? Oh no, Mother.'

I was confused, wracking my brains to try and work out when I might have said something. Had something slipped out? Who had I been talking to? Surely Cecilia would not have reported me. I felt sick to the bottom of my stomach.

'Yes. Do not compound the offence of complaint with the offence of an untruth. It does not behove a member of this Community, particularly one so new, to be ungrateful for the food that the good Lord feels fit to put on our table.'

Shaken and tearful, I left her office. I went and sought out Sister Clemence. Luckily she knew the answer.

'Oh dear, you must be more careful what you write home.'

Of course: writing home one day and a bit stuck for things to say (the life was so bizarre, it was difficult to find anything to write about that my family would understand), I made a joke about the food. All letters had to left outside the Mother Superior's office unsealed. Stupidly, I hadn't taken on board the implication of leaving them open – she obviously read them all. I was much more careful in future.

I soon came unstuck in the matter of clothes too. When I went to be measured for my postulant's dress, I hadn't realised I was going to have to undress down to my underwear. There I was, standing with the most fearsome Sister Julia glaring at me, as I took off my sensible skirt and blouse and revealed the most lacy black bra and knickers.

'I think a visit to the underwear section of the local department store is in order young lady, don't you?' she said. Blushing, I nodded.

'Totally, totally inappropriate.'

This was my introduction to Sister Julia and it set the tone for our future encounters.

Unfortunately it was also Sister Julia that I ran into literally one night, when, in a quick dash to the loo, I came across her dressed in my 'old night attire', which I was dutifully wearing out. Unfortunately being a twenty-something girl at the end of the Fifties, my old night attire was a short black 'baby doll' nightie with black frilly knickers. The next day I received a note from Mother Sarah Grace,

> *Dear Catherine Mary,*
>
> *I am writing to remind you of the Community rule that your long navy blue dressing gown must be worn at all times outside your bedroom at night.*

Because I still had to wear my habit, at this stage my postulant's dress and veil, I could never really have a break from being in the Community. However, I did on occasion dash off down the road for a swim. Public beaches in Hastings were forbidden – the sight of a nun stripping into her costume was deemed far too interesting for the sort of people who frequented the town beaches, but we were allowed to swim in a pool at a local school.

I was very struck by this on the first occasion I ventured out. I had been at the Mother House for a month and I was beginning to forget that there was a world outside the convent. For this reason when Cecilia suggested that a few of us postulants and novices take a trip to the cinema, I was overcome with both excitement and fear.

We first had to ask Mother Sarah Grace's permission. As with our visits to the library (we were allowed to go and borrow books as long as we brought them to her for her approval; nothing of an 'emotional nature' was permitted), we were allowed to go if the requested film was deemed 'suitable' i.e. that there would be nothing too excitable or corrupting for us.

We sat around and debated what we dared ask to see.

'Well, I reckon we could get away with *The Bridge on the River Kwai*,' Cecilia said.

'How about *A Farewell to Arms*?' Novice Eve volunteered.

'Rock Hudson and Jennifer Jones?' Cecilia looked incredulous.

'It's Hemingway.'

'Exactly. It's a love story.'

'Yes, but is she going to know that?'

'Her whiskers can sniff out a romance from a mile away,' I joined in. Cecilia tried again.

'There's always *The Bridge on the River Kwai*?'

We sat in silence pondering. Then a novice called Christina piped up, 'I'd love to see *Funny Face*.'

'Yeah, and I'd love to see *Gunfight at the O.K. Corral*,' Eve said.

'Cecilia, I dare you to go and ask for *The Prince and the Showgirl*,' I begged.

We laughed and then fell silent again. Cecilia sighed.

'OK, I'll go and ask if we can see *The Bridge on the River Kwai*.'

As Cecilia had predicted, *The Bridge on the River Kwai* was deemed respectable, so with our Mother Superior's blessing, and having persuaded Sister Clemence to give us a lift, the four of us piled into the Morris Minor and lurched off into Hastings at 30mph in second gear in the centre of the road.

It was only when we arrived in the municipal car park and had to climb out of the car that it hit me – I was in a habit with a veil over my head and a large cross around my neck. Not only that, I was with a whole group of habits. I suddenly felt very self-conscious. I noticed a couple of young men looking at us and smirking. I knew what they were thinking, or at least I thought I did. It was only until very recently that I would have been thinking the same thing myself. And I realised that a group of four young nuns walking through the town and going into the cinema and sitting down and watching a film would stick out. People would look at us and probably make jokes about which film we were going to see. *The Prince and the Showgirl?* – cue laughter. If I did anything out of character in my habit – laugh loudly, trip up, cry – it would be noticed and judged that bit more than if it had been me in my ordinary clothes. And that was the worse thing of all; I felt as if no one would see me any more. They wouldn't be able to get past my habit. I sat in the cinema, in the welcome anonymity of the dark, and silent tears fell down my face. I wasn't crying for the poor PoWs in the film; I was mourning my old life and my old self, and my old freedom to be me.

It all came to a head on Good Friday. I was serving the traditional fish pie lunch. The Sisters were all sat in solemn silence as befits such a key, dark day in the Church's calendar – the day of our Lord's crucifixion. I was placing the dishes of pie at even spaces along the long wooden table, but before I could get the plates in front of the Sisters, Sister Felicity had grabbed an enormous helping and was spooning it straight on to her placemat. I looked along the line. Everyone had seen, I saw a few smothered smiles and then I saw shoulders shaking as they tried to hide their amusement. I couldn't help myself any longer. I burst out laughing and dropped the plate I had been holding. I had been so buttoned up for so long, my shoulders were heaving and the more I tried to stop, the more this irrepressible laughter just kept on going. It was a visit from the giggle bug you only get at the most inappropriate times – funerals, classrooms, doctors' waiting rooms, just when you shouldn't. In fact the more you shouldn't, the more difficult it is to stop.

'Catherine Mary, would you please leave the refectory until you can control yourself,' Mother Sarah Grace said firmly.

I hurried out and took some deep breaths in the fresh air, laughter gone, shame taking its place.

So why then, why did I stay? The answer lay in the chapel. I loved the chapel: the vaulted ceiling, the clear glass windows letting in shafts of light, the incense in the services that rose to the rafters and then descended again, cloaking us in the scent of the heavens.

On Easter Sunday I sat in the service silently in prayer, and I was filled with a kind of ecstasy. I started thinking about how I had started the journey, and I realised that it was the anniversary of my father's death. I still missed him, but being in this place had brought me closer to him and to our eternal Father. I felt the division between this world and the next evaporating with the holy incense.

There were two things happening for me at the convent. On one level, I was being moulded, conditioned, processed into a way of life and being. This required me to give up something of myself. But although I was struggling with it and railing against it, I was aware that, as with all things that are worth having, something has to be given up. Because what I was gaining was something on a much deeper level: something more fundamental. I was being given the opportunity to form a profound relationship with God. Religious life demands that however busy our day, we stop and pray five times a day. This means that we are in a constant dialogue with God. In any relationship with a partner, you have to be in constant communication: sometimes talking, sometimes in silence, but always thinking of the other; in this way you get to know each other, your relationship isn't static. You have good days and bad days but it is dynamic and alive. I knew that I wanted to have God at the centre of my life. Nothing was more important, and this habit and this life gave me both the permission and the opportunity to do so. And on this Easter Sunday, for the first time, I was profoundly grateful that this was so.

When you take those life vows and become a Sister, you put on a wedding ring to signify your consecration to Christ. In my first 40 days at the convent I had come to realise that I had started my courtship. My relationship with God had gone to a new level and I was learning more about Him, and it was the most joyful experience. I had a sense that I was on a journey and I had found myself in the right place at the right time.

I had come home.

CHAPTER THREE
OBEDIENCE

When Mother Sarah Grace told me I was to spend my first six weeks at the Mother House digging up the rhododendrons I was a bit perplexed. The Mother House had a nursing home attached to it, and I had presumed that because I had told them I wanted to become a nurse, I would start off working there. However it seemed she thought I would be better employed digging up some of the roots of the huge bushes that lined the driveway. I only hoped my newly mended ankle would be up to it.

My one consolation was that my digging companion was to be Sister Rachel. I had observed Sister Rachel from afar. She looked like fun. This impression was confirmed one night when, waiting outside the bathroom for my turn for a bath, I heard peals of laughter coming from inside. Within minutes Mother Sarah Grace was hurrying down the corridor and banging on the door.

'Sister Rachel, Sister Rachel, open this door immediately! Who have you got in there?'

The laughing stopped. There was silence.

'Sister Rachel, I demand that you open the door. Now!'

There was the sound of dripping water and padding feet. The lock turned and the door opened a crack to reveal a dripping-wet Sister Rachel, wrapped in a towel and holding a book.

'I'm sorry, Mother, but it's that Lent book you gave us to read. Chapter Two is so hilarious.'

(It was quite amusing, but I thought hilarious was pushing it a bit.)

The Reverend Mother looked stunned.

'Really, Sister Rachel! I do not think the bath is an appropriate place to contemplate a spiritual text.'

And with that our Reverend Mother turned on her heels and left. Sister Rachel winked at me, closed the door and locked it again.

So we started digging. Six hours a day. It was dirty, hard work and it wasn't long before the old question was popping out of my mouth.

'But why? Why are we doing this? Why are we spending our time digging up perfectly good bushes?'

'Ours is not to question, Catherine Mary,' Sister Rachel said wryly.

'But this is ridiculous. There's a nursing home up there filled with people whom we could really help.'

'Obedience, Catherine Mary, obedience. This is where we are required to start doing things that are asked of us with a gracious spirit, even if we can't see a logical reason behind it. These are the first steps towards giving ourselves to God and one another.'

I looked at her to see if she was being serious. She looked like she was. Sister Rachel continued.

'Yes, I think you may find obedience the most challenging of the three vows. It certainly has been in my experience anyway.'

'Oh.' I was a little surprised.

'Have you ever heard the stories about how the Benedictines used to ask their novices to water twigs?'

'No.'

'Well, they did; to teach them obedience over rational thought, I presume; something about releasing the soul from the ego. They might still do it actually.'

I had to stop and think for a moment.

'Gosh!' I said, 'that's extraordinary. But surely they run the risk of turning us into unthinking children. What about individual choice and responsibility and our own relationship with God?'

'Catherine Mary, I am going to ask you a question and I want you to think hard before you answer it.'

I nodded.

'If you are looking for the truth, what do you think you have to have above all else?'

I thought, but in the absence of anything more profound I said, 'An absolute determination to find it?'

She shook her head.

'No. To find truth you have to have the ability and willingness to admit you may be wrong. Truth is based on listening to those around you, this is the only way to grow closer to God.'

That set me thinking, and gradually, as the days went by, I began to wonder whether there was method in the Reverend Mother's madness. By putting me in such close proximity to Sister Rachel and making us share such an arduous task, we were bonding. Sisters come in all psychological shapes and sizes, but Sister Rachel was a clever choice for me. She was fun, open and genuine. I wanted to know her story and she was happy to tell me, and suddenly the days of hard labour started to fly past.

Sister Rachel had spent the Second World War working in the East End, firstly at the London Hospital in Whitechapel and then at the Mission House in Poplar. Her stories were painted against a background of fear. She told me how when she thought of Whitechapel, she tasted dust.

'It used to get in my mouth, in my ears, up my nose. It was all the debris from the bombing, I think. I was very lucky I was on my day off the day the hospital was hit. My best friend was a nurse on the same ward and one minute she was tucking up the men in bed and the next minute there was an enormous explosion. She said it was followed by a strange silence. Then a patient said, "Hold on, Sister. Don't move until I've found a light."

'He found a torch, she turned round and there was the most enormous hole in the wall. Just a gaping hole, where seconds before there'd been two beds. Imagine. A terrible thing for two of your patients to be there one minute and poof, gone the next!'

She paused, then went on, 'Actually I had the only cigarette I've ever had just a few weeks later during another bombing raid.'

Sister Rachel had a day off and went to visit an old aunt in South London. On her way back she got caught in a bombing raid while on the Tube somewhere around St Paul's. The packed Tube train stopped at the station and the doors opened. Rachel started to get anxious. She was due back at the Mission House at 10 p.m. If she got out and ran, she might just make it back in time. If she waited for the train service to start again she could be there all night. She was standing next to two rather attractive naval officers. 'Excuse me, I wonder whether you could be so kind? I really need to get out of here,' she said. They grinned and picked her up and carried her over the heads of the passengers, out of the train, and pushed passed the wardens, shouting 'Sorry, emergency!'. The wardens were so stunned they waved them past and suddenly the three of them were standing in the street, with bombs falling all around. 'We watched as the planes flew low over London and the fires burned around St Paul's Cathedral. We even shared a cigarette. It was the most destructive and yet the most beautiful thing I have ever seen.'

'Weren't you scared?'

'No, I wasn't. I knew God had a lot more He wanted me to do.'

I was impressed by Sister Rachel's quiet faith and yet puzzled by how such a feisty young woman came to find herself tucked away in the cloisters, so one day I asked her about her vocation.

'I felt God calling me to the Community when I was quite young,' she said, 'really, it was all to do with my mother's death.'

Sister Rachel's mother had been fragile for as long as she could remember. One day, walking home from visiting her in hospital, Rachel's father stopped on the corner of their road and said, 'This is it for your mum. She's never going to get any better. You've got to be brave and face it: Mum is going to die.'

For the next few years, with her father at work, and being an only child, Sister Rachel had to work hard at school as well as nurse her fading mother. The district nurse taught her how to wash her, measure out her medicine and prepare her for injections. It was hard watching her mother get weaker but Rachel's grief was tempered by the fact that she could help her mother. In those precious last years together, Rachel and her mum grew very close. Then, when Rachel was 13, her mother finally died. Again the wise district nurse helped Rachel by letting her help lay out her mother's body. Rachel helped wash and dress her. It was an experience that left a deep impression on her.

That summer she was sent to stay with her penfriend in Sweden. When Rachel got back, her father greeted her with the news that he had remarried. For Rachel, this marriage came completely out of the blue and seemed so soon after her mother's death. Indeed, she felt she was no longer welcome in her own home.

Touched by her plight, Rachel's head teacher paid a visit to the local hospital and managed to get Rachel accepted to train as a cadet nurse much earlier than usual. It was while she was training that she found herself working alongside a woman who regularly visited the Community and she took Rachel first to church and eventually to visit the Mother House.

'From the moment I arrived, I knew I had found my new home, I had found the right place.'

Sister Rachel smiled at me.

'I hope it will come to feel that way for you too, Katie.'

I was touched. I hadn't heard my Christian name spoken for a long time and I didn't know quite what to do with myself. So I dug just a little bit harder at the rhododendron roots and watched my tears fall into the hole.

At the end of the six weeks I was called back to Mother Sarah Grace's office.

'Catherine Mary, I have decided it is time you were introduced to the nursing home.'

I was delighted. Ever since the day I helped Sister Dorothy make Old Sue comfortable, I had thought

I would like to join the nursing profession in some capacity (while not being convinced about the vision of myself as a Sister).

The nursing home was in a house further up the drive. There were three floors, with a kitchen in the basement, a long refectory, an office and a communal visiting room on the ground floor. Upstairs there were two wards and then on the top floor there were some private rooms. We had about 30 patients. They were mainly elderly people who needed nursing care but did not have much money, but there were also a few younger patients who needed respite care, and then a few who were chronically or terminally ill. The Community wanted to provide good-quality care for people who otherwise could not have afforded it.

The first thing that struck me was how hard the work was. The hours were long – we started with early prayers at 6 a.m., and then had a Communion followed by breakfast. The day shift at the nursing home lasted from 8 a.m. to 8 p.m., with a couple of hours off duty either in the morning or the afternoon. A period of night duty would involve 14 nights in a row working from 8 p.m. to 8 a.m. There was, though, some recognition that this was tough. After my first night shift, I was enormously touched to find a full kettle and some biscuits left outside my room. Mother Sarah Grace had put them out for me when she got up. Unlike most of the others, I'd had no nursing training and so I was given the most basic jobs – cleaning the equipment, making the beds, washing the commodes. After six weeks on commode duty, Mother Sarah Grace called me into her study.

'Catherine Mary, I know you have been working very hard on the commodes. It's time to give you something different ... from now on you will be in charge of washing the dentures.'

I really didn't find this an improvement. In fact it took me a while to get used to the intimacy of nursing. We had a very high standard of care towards our patients. Much of my time was spent clipping nails, brushing hair and cleaning teeth. Our incontinent patients were kept scrupulously clean. We gave bed baths every day. All the patients had little bells beside their beds that we answered immediately. One old patient, an old Sister of St John's, just used to tap her wedding ring on the metal side of her bed to get attention; the sound lives with me to this day. Then there was Miss Wittering. She was a sweet old lady who loved her cups of tea, but she always spoke in code. The novice's habits at that time were bright blue and she used to beckon me over and whisper in my ear, 'Hyacinth, darling.'

I was confused until one day I realised that this was her way of asking for the bedpan. She always used to wake up in the middle of the night and ring her bell and shout 'Hyacinth, darling', disturbing all the rest of the patients. I worked out that I could stop her from waking up the rest of the ward by creeping over and whispering in her ear, 'I'm going to make a cup of tea, Miss Wittering, would you like one?' She'd be instantly awake and nod vigorously. 'I'll bring you a hyacinth first, shall I?' Again there would be a vigorous nod. In this way the other patients got a good night's sleep.

Miss Wittering was also very useful because of her crossword skills. Sister Joan was in charge of the night wards at the time. She was a lovely gentle soul, but definitely a creature of habit. One of our patients had worked for the *News of the World* and was sent a complimentary copy every Sunday. Once he'd read it, the newspaper would be laid on the floor downstairs to stop people slipping. Sister Joan could be seen peering down at the copy, with her hands on her hips, tutting and giggling, totally engrossed. She absolutely refused to do the rounds until she'd had three cups of tea and finished the crossword. This was fine if the crossword was easy, but sometimes she got stuck and sometimes I got stuck too; and then we all got behind, which wasn't good, not least because the patients were late having their medicines. All was resolved when I realised I could take Miss Wittering a cup of tea and ask to have a look at her paper. She'd invariably have completed the crossword and I could go back to Sister Joan and miraculously suggest the answers.

'My child, you are a genius!' Sister Joan would chuckle.

Working in the home I also saw a different side to our Reverend Mother. There was a woman in one of the top rooms whom I dreaded visiting. Mrs Gidding made me nervous; the flesh was weak but the spirit still fearsome. She watched me closely, and of course the more she watched, the more nervous I became, and the more I fumbled about. One day I was struggling with her bed, when Mother Sarah Grace walked in and said, 'Hello, Mother, and how are you feeling today?'

'Well, it took you long enough to come and ask,' Mrs Gidding replied.

I looked up, confused. Had I imagined it or had she just called her 'Mother'?

Mother Sarah Grace turned to me and said, 'Catherine Mary, have you been introduced to my mother?'

'Yes. Yes, I have, Reverend Mother.'

I felt myself blushing and tried to make myself invisible as the conversation continued.

'And why didn't you come and see me last night?' Mrs Giddings demanded.

'I was in London visiting the Mission House and the train got back late.'

'Well, what makes you think I want to see you now? I don't. Go away.'

Mother Sarah Grace bowed her head and with an air of resignation, rolled her eyes at me and walked out. This strong, disciplined, authoritative woman could also be a chastened, humble daughter.

As I got to know the patients, and overcame my inhibitions, I began to really enjoy the work. There seemed to be something special about caring for these people who, at the end of their lives, were vulnerable. It felt like God's work and I felt a humility and a wave of love for them – they had been somebody's child, survived wars, and had lived long and full lives. I felt they should be treated with respect.

There were some heartbreaking moments too. A few of our patients were younger and were staying with us because they were chronically ill. Cathy was in her thirties and crippled with multiple sclerosis. A 'healing' woman used to visit her and eventually persuaded her that she should go to a special healing service in a church close by. As the day approached Cathy got very excited. She kept talking about what she was going to do once she had been healed. I was concerned that she was putting too much faith on the service working a miracle. It's not that I thought that the service couldn't work or that miracles don't sometimes happen, but I believe they don't always happen. It's an important distinction and I felt the healer was raising Cathy's hopes too high. Anyway, the day arrived and she went off in a special ambulance in great spirits. We all went out to wave her goodbye and wish her luck. But when she arrived back in the evening, she was still in her wheelchair. The healer, who was pushing her, was bright and breezy but I didn't like the look on Cathy's face.

'I've told Cathy that these things can take time. All you need is faith, isn't that right, Sister?' the healer said.

I didn't know what to reply. I felt as if I had been put on the spot and if I agreed and Cathy didn't get better she'd think that it was because she didn't have enough faith. I just didn't know whether God worked in that way or, indeed, whether anyone had the right to claim that was the way God worked. So although Cathy was looking up at me imploringly, I felt I had to be honest.

'I'm just at the beginning of my journey towards God,' I said. 'I believe he does indeed move in mysterious ways and I cannot claim to know how miracles work and indeed I'm not sure I will ever be able to claim that I do. But I hope with all my heart that you improve and find a greater peace, Cathy.'

Cathy looked crestfallen and that day marked the start of a rapid decline in her health. It was as if she gave up hope and lost the will to live. She died just a year later. It upset all of us greatly and was terrible to witness. No matter how much I know that if there was a mistake anywhere it was more likely to do with the faith invested in the healing service, I still couldn't help but blame myself a little for Cathy's decline.

There was also a man in his early sixties who had multiple sclerosis and was paralysed from the neck down. He had the mind of a grown man in the body of a baby; we changed his nappy, fed him with a spoon and wiped his nose. He had fixed ideas how he wanted everything done, and however way I did it, it was never to his satisfaction. As I leaned over him I had to brace myself for a running barrage of criticism. Sometimes I walked off the ward in tears. After a particularly difficult day I was walking back to the Mother House, trying to hide my tears, when I was spotted by Sister Rachel. She saw my distress and I had to explain. She paused for a minute, then took my arm and, walking me slowly back to the Mother House, told me a story.

'At the time of the Second World War, Whitechapel had a large Jewish community and the London Hospital had a special Jewish ward. We even had a kosher kitchen. There was a young rabbi in the ward who was dying from cancer. In those days there was no treatment, just some pain relief given every four hours that involved a lot of morphine. One night I was on duty and the rabbi kept asking for a bedpan. In those days we didn't just hand them the pan and leave them to do the job. We had to silently move the screens around their bed to give them privacy, and then we had to hold the pan for them and clean them up afterwards. Poor man! He had to ask me for the pan over and over again. But just as morning came and I went to him one last time, as I knelt at his bedside, he put his hands on my head and said, "Dear Sister, I have asked you to come how many times tonight? And every time you have come with a smile. Bless you, my child."

'A few weeks later he was dead, but I realised how important the way you behave is, to come with a smile, to have compassion. This is the work, the test, our vocation. This is truly what God is asking from us.'

She put her arm around me and reached into the pocket of her habit.

'Here, have a humbug,' she said and handed me a sweet. That afternoon I felt her compassion towards me too.

Later on that month my difficult patient went on his annual pilgrimage to Lourdes. A specially prepared ambulance, known as the 'jumbulance' arrived to drive him all the way through France. When he came back he seemed much better, at peace with himself. I realised it was his own terrible inner demons that had been attacking me and I was glad that God had given me the inner strength to carry on nursing him.

In my novitiate classes, learning about the history of the Community, I realised that this question of obedience is a constant tension in the religious life. When is God calling us to obey and when is He calling on us to stand firm? It is a question of judgement and I was struck that when I was taught about the early history of the Community how Mother Superiors themselves could be rather disobedient. Indeed, Sister Mary Jones was anything but obedient. Right from the start she objected to the interference of the male Master, the Reverend Gipps. As happens in many families, Mother kept trying to overrule Father and vice versa, but unlike in a real family, there was a governing body that both could run to in order to adjudicate. Mary Jones found that she couldn't dismiss the nurses whom she felt were proving unsuitable, without Reverend Gipps's permission. Anyone whom she tried to 'let go', Reverend Gipps supported.

She complained that his pressure to employ more probationers had led them to become disobedient. The Reverend claimed that, on the contrary, the probationers were unruly because Mary Jones was 'unjust and unmerciful', and treated them as overgrown children. He said that Mary Jones didn't allow him to investigate whether the nurse was in the right or wrong. He thought that she had caused the disciplinary problems by setting such a bad example herself. He said that the Mother Superior must always defer to the Master, 'where the law of nature places him, over and not under a female officer'. Gipps insisted that any alteration in the rules was 'a course of policy which must terminate in substituting a woman for a man in the government of a house: a result of which, I believe, would speedily leave no house to be governed'.

Mary Jones was having none of this. She threatened to resign unless Gipps was replaced and Gipps threatened to resign unless Jones was replaced. Mary Jones responded by asking the governing council to abolish the post of Master and appoint her as the ultimate authority in the Community. She was so indispensible and capable that the Board of Governors agreed not only to remove the troublesome Reverend Gipps, but also gave her a seat on the governing board. This was perhaps the first time that a woman had managed to sit on such a committee with the same authority as men.

However, a couple of years later Sister Mary stretched her lack of obedience too far when she asked that the

Sisters be allowed to appoint a chaplain of their own choosing. In reality Mary Jones and many of her Sisters were longing to become a more strictly and overtly religious order, closer to their Catholic counterparts. But in the 1860s anti-Catholic feeling was still very strong. The Bishop agreed to her request as long as the chaplain did not hear Confession and the Sisters did not take the vows of poverty, chastity and obedience. Sister Mary Jones insisted that these ministrations would be in no way compulsory and only for those Sisters who wanted them. She wrote: 'I am an old woman now and I have seen this longing for the religious life spreading widely and deeply among the daughters of our beloved church.'

Her best friend, Florence Nightingale, waded in, 'Tell them what you want is not a Committee of inquisition but a simple chaplain. *Pricipios Obsta* [sic] – oppose any such ecclesiastic domination.'

But the new Bishop of London would not allow it and wrote to Mary Jones: 'You must be ready to sacrifice your own individual tastes and wishes when those placed over you in the Lord advise you should make the best of the circumstances in which you find yourselves.'

It was not the response that Sister Mary Jones was looking for and she resigned, stating, 'We must demand the right to regulate our own inner life'.

She left, taking six of the eight Sisters with her, and, despite offers to take up a leading role in the London hospitals, she set up a Sisterhood of district nurses and a chronic care hospital which is still flourishing today, independently from the Community of St John.

I felt this spirit of rebellion keenly during my first Christmas at St John's House. As the festive season approached, I became acutely aware of what I was missing in the outside world, not least what my family would be up to at my old home. Edward coming back from work with a tree, the party at the local Labour building just round the corner with dodgy rum punch which always ended in a singalong round the piano and a crazy mix of carols and 'We'll Keep the Red Flag Flying', Elsie and my nephews and nieces coming round. The men would all retreat to the Gloucester Arms while the women prepared lunch and would be back in time for the Queen's Speech. My grandmother decorating the Christmas pudding with a sprig of holly and too much lit brandy and the lethal threepenny pieces she'd hidden inside, with the day culminating in our own family sing-song, 'I Dreamt I Dwelt in Marble Halls', with the harmonium squelching because some uncle had poured beer inside it.

I had been at the Mother House for nine months without a break. However much I was beginning to appreciate it, it was incredibly hard, unrelenting work. The half day a week that we were given off only started at 2.30 p.m. I was starting to feel really tired. Not the sort of tiredness that could be sorted with one night's good sleep, but a more profound, deeper tiredness that seemed to be sinking right down into my bones.

Of course at Christmas we gave most of the support staff a few days off, which meant that we all had to work especially hard. We also had more religious services to fit in. So, after a full 12-hour shift on Christmas Eve we had to stay up for Midnight Mass and then we had to get up to sing Christmas carols on the stairs at the nursing home at 5.30 a.m. My 'Ding Dong Merrily on High' was sung through gritted teeth. I have no idea if the patients appreciated it. Then we started a full day of the normal nursing duties punctuated by a large Christmas lunch. By the start of the Boxing Day shift my goodwill to all men was practically non-existent. 'How on earth am I going to survive a lifetime of this?' was the question I kept asking myself through that first festive season.

You can imagine, therefore, how much I was looking forward to the day of silence and contemplation that was planned a few weeks later. Part of the religious life involves periodically taking time out for retreat. This is a time of specific length spent away from one's normal life in order to connect at a deeper level with God. I was told I was allowed to spend my day in any way that I chose, as long as it was solitary and in silence, and I was back in the chapel for evening prayer.

I had been gazing at that enchanted forest outside my bedroom window for a while and I was determined to grab my chance. After my silent lunch I headed off into the trees. It was beautiful. London girl that I was, the closest that I had got to a forest was a small copse on

Hampstead Heath. I found myself surrounded by peace and darkness, as if I was the only person alive. I heard my footsteps snapping twigs underfoot, the odd bird singing, a rustle as I disturbed a woodland creature. With this freedom I decided to go off the path, to wander and see where the Holy Spirit took me.

In my reverie I remembered the film of Disney's *Snow White* that I had seen as a child and I half expected to see a small cottage complete with seven singing dwarfs on their way home. I wasn't afraid, but I felt that God was with me, taking me on a magical journey out of the intensity which at times felt overwhelming to something free and more basic, the beauty of creation. It was easy to forget God's natural world when I spent so many hours in man-made buildings. As I pondered these things I suddenly remembered the time: I had to be back at five o'clock for evening prayers. I felt an instant sense of panic. Where was the path? I started to head in what I thought was the right direction, but I only seemed to be getting deeper and deeper into the forest and the light was fading fast.

I imagined the Sisters gathering, an empty space on my pew. The forest didn't seem so benign now, and I had an image of Hansel and Gretel and their breadcrumbs being eaten. 'Dear Lord, show me the way,' I prayed. Shadowy thoughts started to enter my head. Perhaps I hadn't been guided by the Holy Spirit but something darker? An internal debate started with one voice saying,

'What's the worst that could happen? It was a genuine mistake, so you miss Evening Prayer.' But another voice was telling me off for my stupidity, my willfulness, my arrogance in thinking I could find my own way. There is only one path. 'Dear God,' I prayed. 'Please let me find the path. I promise I will never stray from the path again.' Into my head strayed a paragraph about those who chose the religious life from the rule of St Benedict: 'It is love that impels them to pursue everlasting life; therefore, they are eager to take the narrow road of which Jesus says "Narrow is the road that leads to life". They no longer live by their own judgement, giving in to their whims and appetites; rather they walk according to another's decisions and directions, choosing to live in monasteries.'

I realised however much I was irritated by the rules of the convent, deep down I still really wanted to conform, I wanted to be part of the Community and I wanted to make it work. I don't know how long I walked in what seemed like circles, but suddenly I saw the path in front of me. Filled with relief, I quickly headed out. In front of me was the Mother House and a group of Sisters walking towards me.

'Where have you been? We have all been worried about you, you silly girl.' Sister Julia seemed to relish the opportunity to scold me.

I was taken into Mother Sarah Grace's study, where I was given a lecture about missing prayers, the selfishness of worrying the Community, how I must never do this again. I apologised and she could see I was genuinely shocked and upset.

'I'm so, so sorry. I was lost; I wandered from the path. I will never do it again,' I said.

Her face softened. 'Yes, I can see. You look frightened. I'm sure you have learnt a lesson. Sometimes we have to wander from the path in order to see how important it is for us to stay there.'

I nodded.

'Christ himself spent 40 days in the wilderness. You've just had an afternoon and yet how powerful just an afternoon can be. It might be useful to spend some time thinking about that. God sometimes allows us to wander, so we can make our own decision whether to come back. And it seems you have come back. Which leads me to something I have been wanting to talk to you about. Catherine Mary, we have decided that if you wish, you should proceed to the next stage: to your clothing, to becoming a novice. We think you are ready. Is that what you would like?'

I was overcome with joy. I hadn't realised how much I really wanted to take the next step until this moment.

'Oh yes, Mother, thank you.'

A few years later I watched *The Sound of Music*. In the opening scene the postulant nun, Maria, is so caught up in the joy of singing on top of a mountain that she misses evening prayers. I chuckled and felt the truth of it.

Was I Julie Andrews? And as soon as I had the thought, I realised I was not: I had taken a different path. I was glad that Mother Sarah Grace hadn't banished me to be a nanny in the outside world, but instead had had faith, as I had done at that moment, that I was on the right path.

CHAPTER FOUR

RELEASED INTO THE WILD

Sometimes people ask me what comes first – do I see myself primarily as a nun, or as a nurse and a midwife? But the question itself is misguided. To me they are inseparable. My life as a nun and my life as a nurse both come from my belief in God. I am called to do both; my vocation is to put God at the centre of my life and express this in the world by being a nurse and a midwife. This really started to become clear in my second year at the Community.

Very early one frosty winter's morning in 1960, I found myself putting on my royal blue novice habit for the first time. 'Hyacinth, darling,' I said to myself as I smoothed down its voluminous folds. I had been given it, freshly blessed, at Compline the night before. Reverently, I carried it back to my room and lay it on the chair next to my bed. All night I kept waking up and looking at it nervously. Would the clothes ever feel like a perfect fit or would I feel like I was dressing up? In the end I gave up on sleep and spent the rest of the night on my knees in the dark in silent prayer.

Becoming a Sister is a long process. It takes longer than getting a university degree. In fact it's the equivalent of starting at university and staying there until you have completed a PhD. And like being at university, at various points you are assessed and examined, and only allowed to proceed to the next stage with the permission of the Mother's Council. It's not an automatic process. Only a few are chosen to go through what's known as 'the Narrow Gate'. (Taken from a passage of Matthew's Gospel, 'Enter through the narrow gate, for wide is the gate and broad is the road that leads to destruction, and many enter through it. But small is the gate and narrow the road that leads to life, and only a few find it'.)

Despite it's rather cosy, Women's Institute-sounding name, the Mother's Council was very serious. It was made up of the Mother Superior and four other senior Sisters and they met periodically to discuss the most important Community matters. At some point, I must have come up in 'Community matters' and been deemed ready to be invited to become 'clothed', which is the term they used to describe becoming a novice. Although Mother Sarah Grace never said it, I had the feeling that she liked and understood me, and despite her severe, devout manner she was capable of genuine love for us. I already felt a deep respect for her but there were others in the Community whom I felt might have made a different judgement about me, because there was judging in the convent, particularly from the older generation who had lived through even more exacting and severe regimes. That night I prayed that I would not let Mother Sarah Grace down.

As the light began to peep through my curtains, I got up and started to get dressed. My anxious prayers seemed to have been justified when I pulled the habit over my head. It was enormous; I looked less holy than wholly comic. It was only later that I discovered that despite going to the bother of measuring you, they only made the habits in one size. However once I'd tied a belt round me and hitched it up a little, I looked a bit more convincing. Then I faced the dilemma of how to tie my new veil – it was just a square of white cloth. 'Dear God, help me,' I prayed, giggling slightly hysterically as I tied various crazy configurations around my head. Eventually I thought I had got it right but when Sister Rachel came in to check on me, she laughed. I had tied my veil so tightly under my chin that I couldn't open my mouth. 'Is that so you can't say "thank you" when the Chaplain puts your new cross round your neck?' she said, undoing it and starting again.

I was clothed as a novice before the usual early-morning Communion service so, as always, the whole Community was there, with only the presence of the Chaplain General signifying that this was a special day. But as I stood and turned to look at the congregation, I noticed an extra face at the back of the chapel. It was my mother. I was astonished: I'd written to her, telling about my journey of faith and that I was going to be clothed, but I never expected her to come and witness it, especially as I was sure she hadn't had a 'road to Damascus' conversion over the whole idea of me becoming a nun. I had prickles down the back of my throat as I struggled with an overwhelming wave of emotion: the realisation of how much I needed her blessing to be able to move on to my new family and my new home. Although it has to be said, she wasn't looking overjoyed; she looked very serious. But I took this as a sign that, whatever her feelings about my entering the religious life, she would support me and that meant all the world to me.

Not long afterwards I was summoned by Mother Sarah Grace and told that an interview had been arranged for me at the local hospital with a view to starting my proper training to become a nurse.

'I tried to persuade them that you could remain living here and commute every day, but they were having none of it.'

There was a pause. I wasn't sure what the Reverend Mother was implying.

'I'm sorry. You are just going to have to live out.'

'Live out?'

'In the nurses' accommodation.'

'Oh.'

I didn't quite know what to say. Mother Sarah Grace obviously thought this was going to be difficult for me.

I found the idea quite exciting. Out, in the real world. No more curtseying, no more lists, no more restrictions from reading books of an 'emotional' nature, no more censored letters; in fact, no more long nighties and knickers with legs. But – much more seriously – it would be the first real test of my vocation. It's one thing being a nun in a convent, that's hardly radical; quite another to be surrounded by temptation and others who have chosen to live a different way. If I still preferred to live a life of poverty, chastity and obedience with God at the very centre, I would have passed a really big test. I was about to be released from captivity; could I survive with my vocation intact? 'Bring it on,' I thought to myself.

But I had no sooner closed the door to the Reverend Mother's study when I was confronted by Sister Julia, who seemed to have been hovering around outside on purpose.

'Just remember if you make a fool of yourself, do it with dignity,' she said and turned on her heel.

What did she mean? That evening I prayed earnestly in the chapel.

Thankfully, after my interview I was accepted for training and some days later a letter arrived from my new nurse tutor at the hospital, complete with a reading list. In order to become a fully trained nurse I had to be awarded a general nurse's certificate. This meant three years' training through a combination of lectures, tutorials, and practical experience on the wards. As well as having to write essays and case studies, I would have to sit exams at the end of each year, which I would have to pass. My Achilles' heel: studying. I had never excelled at school. It dawned on me that not only my reputation, but the reputation of the Community was at stake and I did not feel confident.

However, leaving the Mother House had a surprise bonus. Mother Sarah Grace sent me a note informing me that because of my need to travel quite frequently between the Mother House and the hospital, on my next afternoon off I was to accompany her into Hastings to purchase a vehicle. So a few days later Mother Sarah Grace and I piled into the yellow Morris Minor with Sister Clemence at the wheel, the Reverend Mother of course in the passenger seat, and me in the back, and we set off into town. As we jolted down the drive in second gear Mother Sarah Grace turned to me with raised eyebrows and a twinkle in her eye and said, 'So as you can see, Catherine Mary, we really do need to find a way for you to make your own way back to us from the hospital.'

Before long we lurched into the forecourt of a vehicle dealer. I noticed two men come to the window and stare as three Sisters struggled to get out of a beaten-up Morris Minor. Once free of the car, Mother Sarah Grace unhurriedly and meticulously straightened her habit. It was something of a revelation to witness her outside her natural habitat: she had lost none of her dignity and authority. She stood naturally poised and still, until the dealers realised she was expecting them to come out and greet her. They hastily stubbed out their cigarettes and strode out.

'Hello, madam ... I mean your reverend ... Majesty.'

'Reverend Mother will do, thank you. And you are?'

'Steve. I mean Stephen: Stephen Hawley, Madam Reverend.'

'Good morning, Mr Hawley.'

There was a pause as Mr Hawley looked uncertain what to do next and Mother Sarah Grace looked at him intently.

'Good morning. Can I help you, Reverend Madam?'

'I hope so, Mr Hawley. Our youngest member, Sister Catherine Mary,' she made a graceful gesture and nod in my direction, 'needs some transport and I believe you may be able to help.'

From somewhere inside the folds of her habit she produced a folded newspaper and, holding it out for inspection, pointed at a ringed advert for a white moped. My heart sank. I had presumed that, miracle of miracles, they were going to buy me a car. Goodness knows the Community could do with some new transport. I tried to quash my toddler-like disappointment.

'Yes, Reverend Majesty. You are in luck! Despite massive interest, this little beauty is still available.'

'I doubt if it is luck, Mr Hawley. Now I would be delighted if we could see the vehicle.'

'Yes indeed, Reverend Majesty. Follow me.'

We trooped around the back of the saleroom and there, down the far end, past all the Jaguars and

Rolls-Royces, Fords and Minis, was a row of motorbikes and, finally, tiny mopeds.

'Here we are, Madam Majesty.'

He pointed to a white moped. It was no more than a bicycle with an engine stuck on the side and reminded me of one of my big brother Edward's early purchases, which was affectionately known in the family as 'the hairdryer'.

'Well, it looks very satisfactory, Mr Hawley.'

'Would you to take it for a spin, Reverend Madam?'

There was a delicious pause. I couldn't wait to see what was going to happen next. For a second it actually looked as if she might do it. I didn't trust myself to look at Sister Clemence.

'No, thank you, Mr Hawley. I will have to decline your offer today. But I think it would be wise for Sister Catherine Mary to give it a trial run. Would you be kind enough to lend Sister Catherine Mary a helmet?'

'Yes of course, your Reverence.'

He nodded to his companion, who came back holding a large white bike helmet. Then he stood in front of me looking awkward: he obviously expected me to take off my veil. Without thinking I started to untie it. I heard Sister Clemence gasp and Mother Sarah Grace quickly said, 'No, Sister Catherine Mary. It will not be, and indeed will never be necessary for you to take off your veil. You will put the helmet over the top – I'm sure it will prove big enough.'

It did indeed prove big enough. With great awkwardness, Mr Hawley's colleague helped me to buckle it up under my chin and then they wheeled out the moped. Feeling slightly ungainly I swung my leg over and climbed on to the seat. Mr Hawley showed me how to start it, and suddenly I was off.

It was an absolutely exhilarating feeling. 'Lord forgive me the hairdryer thing,' I chuckled as I spun round the backstreets of Hastings, habit flying, hands gripping the handlebars, head bent low for greater aerodynamics; I felt like Evel Knievel. No car could ever be this much fun, I thought as I hooted my horn at waving children. It was only with a great sense of disappointment that I realised I had gone too far to be seemly and I had to turn back. As I approached the garage I straightened my back, slowed down to a more appropriate pace and glided sedately into the forecourt.

'Well, Sister?' Mother Sarah Grace asked.

During my time with the Community I had been practising my serious face and I used it now.

'I think this will be adequate for my transport, Reverend Mother.'

She examined my face carefully and then turned to Mr Hawley.

'Well, Mr Hawley, it seems that this moped is the answer to our prayers.'

From within the seemingly boundless capacity of her habit, she produced a wad of notes.

'I think you will find this is sufficient.'

Mr Hawley looked surprised. I wondered whether he had the nerve to count his cash in front of the Reverend Mother, but it seems he didn't, and before I knew it I was off again, flying back to the Mother House on the seat of my new moped.

So in the spring of 1960 I started my three years at the hospital. The nurses' home was in the grounds. We each had our own small room, with a bed, a wardrobe and a desk. As soon as I had unpacked my constant travelling companions – the *Daily Guiding Light*, *The Cloud of Unknowing* and my sacred poetry, I felt at home. We were allowed to put up our own pictures. Most of the girls put up posters of fluffy cats or Cliff Richard. I restricted myself to my favourite icon of St John. There was a small kitchen and a communal sitting room that was immediately a hub of cosy jollity.

On the first day I felt rather self-conscious. I stood out somewhat in my habit. This wasn't helped by the prickly reception I got from the nurse tutor. As we went round the class introducing ourselves, she said to me, 'Oh, hello. Perhaps you'll get us all back on the straight and narrow.'

The class laughed and then her smile disappeared.

'Well, Catherine Mary, if you don't mind we won't be calling you Sister here because you are not entitled to be called a Sister here. In this hospital you will have to work to earn that title.'

'Yes, Sister,' I replied, although I could have pointed out that senior nurses were only called Sisters because they were originally all nuns.

'You will have to wash your habit once a week, you know,' she continued. I bristled and my usual attempt to pursue a course of unconditional positive regard failed.

'I do have more than one habit actually, Sister. In fact I think you'll find I have enough to make sure that I will be able to wear a clean habit every day.'

The class was suddenly quiet and I said a prayer for greater patience but I was bristling with her contempt. In our novitiate classes we had been taught the history of our Community, and I knew that the Sisters of St John had played a central role in the transformation of nursing into a profession rather than a disgrace.

Our founder Robert Bentley Todd's aim was to create a rather superior, a pedigree if you like, kind of nurse. In an unusually enlightened approach, Todd decided that the way to do this was to treat the first Sisters of St John the Divine very differently to their peers.

At that time, most nurses worked a 17-hour day and slept in the hospital attics and basements, or in cupboards off the wards. Their bedding was dirty and overrun with rats. They had to shop for their own food and cook it for themselves, eating in the wards. However, the St John's Sisters and nurses were housed in an elegant Georgian mansion in Fitzroy Square, central London and had a housemaid, a housekeeper, a cook and a laundress at their disposal. They went to work early in the morning, but were expected back at St John's House at 11.30 a.m. for dinner and to start their duties again at 2 p.m. They were to do no dishwashing or cleaning and their duties were exclusively looking after the sick. After 12 years' service they were entitled to a pension and they were given a cottage in the country to use when they needed time to recuperate. Tea, sugar and beer was given to the nurses on night duty and regular day trips out were organised for them to Crystal Palace, Kew Gardens and London Zoo.

Each Sister underwent intensive training for two or more years with classes given by the Sisters on hospital management and lectures on medical matters from doctors, who came into St John's House specially. Their moral education was seen as equally important. They had two services a day – morning and evening prayer taken first by the Chaplain and then, as Mary Jones wrested control, by the Mother Superior herself.

Gossip was seen as dangerous. Mother Mary Jones forbade talking at meals except at tea, after which Sisters then had to retire to their rooms and the lights were turned out after half an hour.

A uniform was introduced of a purple-and-white gingham check dress with a black outdoor cloak and bonnet for the nurses and a full habit of blue for the Sisters, covered by a bib and apron. The nurse's cap was intricately pleated and ribboned, while the Sisters had a plain bonnet, tied at the chin with a huge bow. All the dresses had a short train to make sure that no unseemly ankle was shown when they bent over a patient's bed. The nurses had a bronze badge and the Sisters a large silver cross, both of which had an Eagle of St John on them.

At the beginning the nursing was on a very small scale – when it opened in 1848 there were three sisters, seven nurses and two probationers, undertaking a mixture of private nursing for the rich and nursing of the 'deserving poor'. References and baptismal and marriage certificates had to be produced before the patients would be taken on by Mary Jones (she kept a scrupulous eye on the moral compass of her patients as well as her nurses). Funding came from annual donations from the great and good, and a box which was placed outside St John's House, where the grateful poor put what little spare change they might have in return for services rendered.

The Sisters' private work helped fund their charitable work, such as the case of a poor woman in 1852 who was suffering from severe abscesses after giving birth. A nurse was sent out to her morning and evening in all weathers to change her bandages and bedding, and bring her a lunch of beef tea and jelly and eggs, and a glass of porter or wine at dinner. Another nurse was sent to sit nightly with a poor patient who was dying. She stayed for a fortnight with only two and a half hours' rest a night, and when the man died, she stayed with his widow for six more nights, keeping her company and giving her a present of a pair of curtains when she left. And then there was the case of 'Jane' suffering from a very bad 'ether' from which her recovery seemed hopeless and which made her unremittingly 'fidgety'. Due to the excellent care of the St John's nurses who supplied 'every aid and comfort' she was 'by God's blessing restored to health', but not before two of the St John's nurses caught the infection themselves and had to spend the next 16 weeks being nursed back to health at the Mother House.

As word grew about the Sisters' skills, they found it difficult to keep up with demand. The Committee complained, 'The popular idea of a nurse has unhappily become so low that respectable women hesitate to attach themselves to such a lacklustre society.'

The shortage of Sisters was not helped by the high standards being demanded by the Committee – only one in 20 of those who applied were accepted into the Community. Alarmed, the Sisters advertised in *The Times*. I don't know how successful this was, but the great cholera epidemic of 1853 proved to be a turning point for the Community.

Cholera came to British shores via merchant ships at the start of the nineteenth century. The victim's sunken eyes, blue-grey skin and prolonged, agonising death from vomiting and diarrhoea led to a general sense of panic which wasn't helped by the fact that the disease spread so quickly – in six months in 1853, 11,000 Londoners died and no one had any idea what the cause was. In fact the reason why cholera was so deadly was because it was carried by a bacteria that lives in water and the Thames in London was effectively a giant sewer. Once the cholera bacteria had got into the water system, the whole city was at risk. However, the poorest areas were hit the hardest. The city was rife with rumours that the rich were poisoning the poor.

Into this fevered atmosphere stepped the Sisters of St John the Divine. They were given the task of nursing the cholera wards of Westminster Hospital and greatly impressed the medical profession and the public with their caring and yet professional nursing of the suffering. Articles were written in the newspapers, suitable ladies of a high moral character flocked to join them and within a couple of years the Sisters were approached by King's College Hospital and offered a contract to nurse the whole hospital.

Within their first year of taking over King's, the hospital governors spoke of the Sisters' 'gentleness, intelligence, affection, untiring zeal and self-denial'. In 1866 a report in *The Lancet* said 'the nursing by the ladies is the very best that England has ever seen' and the Sisterhood embodied 'intelligence, keenest sympathy and refinement'. Within a year they were awarded the contract to nurse Charing Cross Hospital too. By 1872 they had to turn down offers to take over the nursing in hospitals as far away as Birmingham and Cambridge. Even Florence Nightingale said, after visiting, how pleased she was with the wards, how cheerful and 'right' an appearance they had. The reputation of the Sisters started to spread across the Channel. Before long they were visited by delegations sent by Napoleon III, the King of Prussia and Tsar Alexander II. The Grand Duke and Duchess of Hesse came in person to see the Sisters, as did visitors from Milan and a number of women from New York, Boston and Philadelphia.

St John's House was the first nurse training institution to be opened in this country, four years before Florence Nightingale set up her own, later more famous, institution down the road at St Thomas's. It was St John's House and not St Thomas's that set the blueprint for the training hospitals like St Bartholomew's and University College Hospital, which were established in the following decades. With this knowledge under my belt, my nursing tutor's hostility seemed a little misplaced. However, she didn't tackle me openly again and I later found out that she'd had a bad experience at a convent school. In fact whenever I encountered a certain coldness from either the staff or patients there was invariably a bad experience in a religious school at the bottom of it, of which unfortunately there seem to be so many.

However, after the first few days everyone seemed to forget my habit and people stopped trying to be polite around me. They even started offering me alcohol and cigarettes, and inviting me to parties; then they stopped again when they realised there was only so far I could and would go. There was a part of me that could never join in, really: that part was given to God.

And that was a really important test. Did I mind that such a joyful part of me was reserved for someone who I couldn't touch or hold? Someone that I couldn't see, and, yes, at the risk of saying the unspeakable, someone who might not even exist? And I didn't. There was no choice or dilemma in my mind. I remembered my anguish at missing my last parish Christmas party and that opportunity to get dressed up, have a drink, flirt with a nice young man. Barely two years had passed and I had no interest in these things; they seemed irrelevant. Coming to the hospital I realised that I had found a meaning and a purpose that transcended having fun. I knew God existed because I was experiencing Him. It is really hard to put into words, but it was something about seeing Him everywhere: in other people, in the world around me. In my solitary moments of prayer I felt Him alongside me, His love and His care. I felt blessed.

Right from the beginning I enjoyed studying. Before we were allowed on the wards we had to spend three months in lectures and tutorials but unlike at school, I was engaged. There seemed to be a real purpose behind what we were learning and I had no problem applying myself. While around me my young companions spent the evenings at parties (and yes, the Sixties had started: I was aware that there was plenty of drug taking and sleeping around, there were even a couple of girls on constant rounds of antibiotics to ward off sexually transmitted disease). I spent my evenings at my desk marvelling at the wonders of the human body, trying to make sense of it and master how to look after it.

It was a happy time for me. I had passed the test, my vocation was safe; indeed I surprised myself with how solid it proved (although I had a feeling Mother Sarah Grace knew I would be safe too, otherwise she would never have let me out into the wild). But saying that, still I enjoyed the camaraderie. It was a lot more fun and relaxed than I was used to. While I didn't join in the parties, I started to find myself in another role – that of priest-confessor. My fellow trainees would pop into my room and talk to me.

What I did miss was the intensity and spiritual companionship of the convent. I only had St John to share my spiritual journey. I tried to keep five daily Offices of Prayer and I turned my room into a mini chapel. I kept a cross in the table drawer beside my bed, which I brought out and propped up; a candle would also be produced and lit. Sometimes I would burn a stick of incense and of course I had my Bible and prayer book. Always aware of what would be happening back at the Mother House and as close to prayer time as possible, I would run back to my room to say my Office – early morning prayers were easy, Compline could be a bit noisy with the partying going on outside my door and of course at lunchtime I couldn't give myself Communion. I wouldn't have had time anyway. As it was I would be running to get there and back to say a few simple prayers, stuffing an egg sandwich in my mouth, robes billowing behind me.

My fellow trainees complained about our workload. I found the opposite: I had much more free time than I was used to. Instead of half a day off a week, I had two whole days. Now I looked forward to a day spent digging the rhododendrons with Sister Rachel: it felt like coming home. One stark reminder of the difference between my fellow trainees and me came over the issue of our salary. At the end of the month there was always lots of talk about how they were going to spend their next month's wages. Clothes, records, vehicles and even houses were being saved up for. 'What are you going to spend your money on, Catherine?' they'd ask. It didn't matter how many times I told them, I didn't see my salary: it was paid directly to the Community and shared out among all of us. They couldn't get their heads around it.

'Gosh, that's hard! Do you really not mind? I couldn't be doing with that,' they'd say, shaking their heads. But I could no longer grasp the concept of money and the whole idea that you might actually only be nursing in order to earn money, and without it you might leave. At the time the opportunity to nurse felt like a gift.

After the first few months of teaching we were deemed ready to be let out onto the wards. From now on our learning would consist of lectures and seminars with practical training on the job. We all waited with eagerness to find out where we were going. There were definite preferences – the men's surgical ward was the most coveted placement. Indeed, all the surgical wards seemed to be preferred to the medical wards. I think this is because generally surgical wards are less physically and emotionally demanding. Patients come in, have their operation and are generally out again quite quickly and in a better state than when they arrived. It's heavy work looking after patients with chronic diseases and, as with so many chronic conditions like kidney disease and emphysema, these patients are never going to get better and that can be really demoralising for the nurses, never mind the patients themselves. I also noticed the nurses preferred working on the men's wards and I think that's because as a young woman, even as a young nun, it's easier to chivvy the male patients on and cheer them up. A smile and a joke can go a long way with the opposite sex.

We were handed our envelopes. I hadn't put in any preference – I wanted it to be God's will where I ended up. I opened up my envelope: my placement was on the men's surgical ward.

'You lucky devil!' the nurses cried.

I was somewhat taken aback. I couldn't remember the last time I'd been called a devil; that's not to say I hadn't felt like one at times. So I'd managed to land myself the plum job. On the first day I came out onto the ward, wearing my habit with an apron over the top. My year in the nursing home had paid off: it felt easy and natural to be there and I was able to start my duties with confidence, especially as there had been such high standards at the Mother House. People's reaction to my Sister's habit was interesting (and mixed). One gentleman who was seriously ill, and in fact didn't have long to live, called me over and said, 'I want to talk to you because you will tell me the truth.'

I actually didn't know what the truth was, but I suspected it was bad. So I went over to the doctor and said, 'Look, you've got to go over and talk to him. He wants and needs to know exactly what you think is going on.'

There was another old gentleman, who had been high up in the Navy, who was seriously ill after heart surgery. He kept telling me he was agnostic but every evening he called me over and talked with me at great length about the meaning of life. One day he opened the drawer beside his bed and got out the Gideon Bible. He opened it at one of the psalms. 'See here, Sister. It says "The fool says in his heart that there is no God".'

He looked terribly sad. Then he took my hand and squeezed it.

'I would like to be able to believe.'

After he had recovered from his surgery, I never saw him again, but for a long time I wondered what had happened to him and whether he ever regained his faith. That's the disadvantage of working in a hospital; if the patient recovers, you never see them again.

It was good to be doing something useful and caring for people, although it was definitely more demanding. Most of the patients in the Mother House had been elderly, long-term residents; in the hospital you had to keep your wits about you and constantly observe your patients. It was acute care and you had to know what to do in an emergency. This was especially true with my next placement, in Accident & Emergency.

The patient who most stays with me was the little two-year-old girl who came in on a hot sunny day. Annie was on holiday with her parents and had run out in front of a car on Hastings High Street. She had suffered terrible injuries and, as was customary in those days, her parents were sent away while we battled to save her. Before they left, I was sent to get her details. I was of course already deeply distressed for Annie and her family, but when her mother told me that her date of birth was 14 November – the same birthday as my little niece – I was really shaken. When I went into the room where she was, I couldn't help but notice her beautiful long blonde hair which, again, was like my niece's. After an hour spent trying to save her, Annie died. The doctor took me aside and said, 'Look, Nurse, somebody has got to ring her parents. I can't do it. Will you do it?'

It was as if my habit gave me an added responsibility, or maybe extra abilities, in the eyes of those around me. I agreed, but I was absolutely dreading it. The parents were staying on a campsite just outside Hastings. I called the campsite phone and the owner answered. I told him that I had some terrible news, and asked him to have the parents ready and, if possible, a doctor for when I rang back a bit later. Half an hour later, her father was waiting for the call. I had to tell him we hadn't been able to save Annie.

When they came back later to the hospital to see her, they thanked us for trying to save her. It was humbling, and as my niece has grown and now has children of her own, I still think that 'this is how old Annie would be now'. Perhaps she would be married and have children of her own. Some patients do penetrate your psyche and stay with you as a living memory and a question. I have prayed many times for her, and for her family. That afternoon as I held her mother I prayed for strength and acceptance and faith in the healing power of God, for her and for me too. I realised my path as a nurse was not always going to be easy. For me the worst moments are when children or young people are irreparably injured. Sometimes I feel haunted. That evening when I turned my bedroom into a little chapel I brought out my book of sacred poems and found William Blake's 'Auguries of Innocence':

> Joy and Woe are woven fine,
> A clothing for the soul divine.
> Under every grief and pine
> Runs a joy with silken twine.

I pondered this verse. Its beauty soothed me except for the nagging thought, where was the joy, where could there be joy in the death of a little girl? Sometimes God doesn't answer me.

There was another day when a young man was brought in. It was his eighteenth birthday. His stepfather had bought him a high-powered motorbike and, egged on by his friends, he'd raced down a hill outside Hastings and come off and landed on his head. He'd suffered terrible internal injuries but he was still conscious. His stepfather kept saying to me, 'I feel so guilty. Why did I do it? Why did I buy it for him? If only I hadn't bought the bike.'

It was terrible to witness. All I could do was say, 'It wasn't you that caused the accident. You're not guilty. Sometimes there are terrible, terrible accidents that are no one's fault.'

A few hours later his stepson died. We sat in a room together as he castigated himself even more ferociously.

'I should never have bought it for him. It's my fault – I've killed him.'

'You haven't killed him. As a parent, that's part of your job. Every parent has to do it: at some point you have to let go, and they have to take responsibility for themselves. This was not your responsibility.'

I'm not sure he was hearing me but there were times when I got the feeling that being a Sister might help. Sometimes the habit was not a barrier but a comfort;

it allowed God into the room and gave permission for a more profound conversation and prayer when often, unfortunately, they were very much needed.

Another young man came in who had been in a car accident. He was badly injured and although we tried to save him, he died within a few hours. His wife, who was in her early twenties (they had only been married for a year) stayed for several hours after he died, talking to me, and we struck up a friendship that lasts to this day. I was so pleased to be invited to her wedding five years later, and I have watched her family grow. Perhaps I am a link to her past and a witness to her present.

It is special work. The shadow side of life and the reality of death and suffering calls for greater reserves of faith and strength. The only way to survive was to keep praying. But I felt useful in that I could perhaps share and ease the pain by being alongside and praying with the patients.

So I was studying hard and really engaging with the work on the wards. I was also getting good marks for my case studies and written work. However, all this was going to be pointless if I didn't manage to pass my exams. I had to get my State Registered Nurse Certificate. This bit of paper was all that really mattered. I was very nervous and only too aware that I had never actually managed to pass an exam. I had Sister Julia's words ringing in my ears that if I did make a fool of myself then I should do so with dignity.

But it was not just about pride: it occurred to me that my vocation was also at stake. At that time the Community of St John was a specialist nursing and midwifery Order. If I failed to get my nursing qualification, then I could no longer remain as part of the Community. The thought was almost unbearable. I realised that there was a difference between being in the outside world safe and contained, as part of a Community with my identity intact, and just being in the outside world alone. I wondered that after only a few years my identity had become so entwined with being a Sister.

We sat in Brighton's Town Hall, in neat rows, all nurses in uniform except for me in my habit. I looked down the rows, spotting the backs of the people I knew – watching Andrew fiddle with his pen and tapping his foot and Fiona being all neat, laying out her pencils. A big clock was ticking loudly on the wall. Everyone had been complaining about how early it was. Not me: I'd been up praying since five o'clock that morning. As I waited to turn over my paper I held on to my cross, fingering the eagle of St John, rubbing it as if a genie might appear and write down the answers for me. I was wildly swinging between the compliant/obedient, 'Wherever you lead me, Lord, I will follow. If this be Your will, then let it be', and then, 'Please God, let me pass. Don't let me fail. Please don't let me down. Please don't let me let You down. Please don't let me let the Sisters down.'

I wasn't making any sense and I realised my faith in the Divine Will was wobbling. In the end I gave up and said, 'Forgive me' and then settled on Julian of Norwich: 'All shall be well, and all shall be well and all manner of thing shall be well'.

'Turn over your papers,' the invigilator said, and then I forgot everything. I was totally engaged and away.

The final hurdle was our Viva. Once again I got on my scooter and rode along to Brighton. I had to go and face a panel and answer questions on practical matters. I remember in particular a rather handsome young doctor in a white coat. I was doing all right, my antiseptic technique went well, but I suddenly started to flounder on infections. I was making it up and I could see he could see I was making it up, and then the bell went.

'Well, Miss Crisp, it seems you have been saved by the bell! Thank you,' he said.

I quickly exited the room.

It was a couple of months before the results came out. I stayed working on the wards and commuting between the hospital and the Mother House. The day before my results were due I was on my way back to the Mother House on my moped and in a world of my own. I was going round a roundabout and a car came straight out in front of me and knocked me flying. The next thing I remember is waking up in a hospital bed, with Mother Sarah Grace sitting beside me. Her eyes were closed deep in prayer. As I waited to try and work out where I was and why, her eyes opened and she stared down at me.

'Catherine Mary, my dear, we have all been so worried about you. You've had a nasty knock, but praise the Lord you will be fine. A few broken bones and bruises, that's all; nothing that won't mend. God be praised.'

Then she bent closer to my face.

'And you passed, my child. You have passed your exams and with flying colours too. You have your State Registered Nurse Certificate and we are all so, so proud.'

CHAPTER FIVE

DELIVERANCE

Mother used to say that when I was born they rang a bell to let the whole world know that another new baby had arrived. Unsurprisingly perhaps, as a child this story had stuck in my mind and rather tickled me. As I got a bit bigger I started to question it – did they really ring a bell for every baby, or was I so special that it was just me? And then as a young teenager I started to think Mother might have got a bit mixed up – she was not the sort to make anything up, but I wasn't aware of bells ringing without a clock or a church service attached.

It was only when I started my midwifery training that I discovered that Mother had indeed heard a bell. But the bell wasn't to announce the arrival of a baby, it was to tell the trainee midwives to get down to the delivery room as fast as possible because there was an opportunity to witness a birth. Before a nurse could qualify as a midwife she had to witness ten deliveries in a hospital and could then work as a midwife conducting deliveries. The bell was rung in the hospital to alert us trainees, so we could drop what we were doing and rush for the labour ward. We'd hopefully have met the mother first in the antenatal clinic, or at least when she arrived in the hospital in the early stages of labour. However, sometimes we didn't have this luxury and just went flying in somewhat apologetically and stood by her side holding her hand, the stranger at the feast.

I absolutely loved every minute of my midwifery training. I hadn't always wanted to be a Sister but as well as wanting to be the actress Vivien Leigh, I had always quite fancied being a midwife. Of course my mother had been a nurse, but I had been more impressed by my much-loved maternal grandmother, who had been one of the women who 'followed the doctor'.

In the old days, when the doctor went to deliver a baby, there would often be a woman following behind on her bike. She would clear up after the delivery and settle the mother. I remembered watching her shoot off on her bike with her big black bag in the basket. She had never been formally trained, but then you didn't have to be in those days: you learned your skills on the job, skills that were passed down from generation to generation.

My grandmother possessed an aura of calm and wisdom, and as I listened to her extraordinary tales of life coming into the world, I longed to be part of those everyday miracles. So when at the beginning of 1963 Mother Sarah Grace announced it was time for me to become a midwife, I couldn't suppress a little squeal. She chose to ignore me and carried on.

'For Part One of your training, we've got you an interview at the General Lying-In Hospital in London.'

'Oh really, Mother, that is wonderful!'

'And for your Part Two you will be going to the Mission House in Poplar.'

She stared at me, as if daring me to look too pleased. I worked hard to stifle my smile. She must have known how much that meant to me. To go back to London, to Poplar, where I had been a parish worker and had so many friends and knew so many people. It felt like a wonderful gift; and of course my real family were just down the road in Camden Town, it would be so easy for me to visit them. It would be another test.

Then as I was leaving the room, she called me back.

'Ah yes, Catherine Mary, one more thing: we hope you will be joined at the General Lying-In Hospital by Sister Cecilia. She hopes to start her training alongside you.'

This time I couldn't contain my joy.

'Oh, Mother, that is truly wonderful news! I have so missed Sister Cecilia.'

It had been nearly four years since Cecilia and I had last shared a room. While I had gone to Hastings Hospital to train as a nurse, Cecilia, who had already got her SRN certificate, had gone to work as a district nurse in the Community's house in Deptford. She had also just taken her life vows and was now a fully-fledged Sister. Although we had bumped into each other at the big gatherings, such as Christmas and Easter at the Mother House, and I had watched her taking her life vows, we had not had a chance to really catch up. So on our first night at the hospital, we enjoyed saying Compline together in my room, and then, by the light of the candle on my home-made altar with a little icon of St John the Divine looking down on us, we started to talk. What Cecilia had to say came as a shock.

'I'm struggling. Really struggling,' she said.

'What do you mean?'

'I don't think I can do this – I don't want to be a midwife. I'm thinking maybe I've taken a wrong turn somewhere.'

I was taken aback. Suddenly I was very aware of the candlelight flickering on Cecilia's gold ring, the ring she was given when she took her final vows to signify her lifelong consecration to Christ.

'But you've just taken your life vows. I mean, isn't that it? You've had the doubt and come through.'

'I know. I thought I'd been through all those struggles with the whole lifestyle and rule – you know what I mean.'

I nodded. Totally.

'It's not God, it's me. I'm not sure about my call to the religious life any more.'

It was shocking to hear such a blunt, honest admission of something that most, if not all, members of the Community had felt at one time or another. I was now gazing at her girdle with its three knots signifying the three vows – poverty, consecrated celibacy and obedience. Cecilia had always seemed so sure of her path.

'What's happened?'

'It's this midwifery. I don't want to become a midwife – I never have.'

'But you love being a nurse.'

'Yes, I do.'

'Well, what's the difference?'

'Well, it's difficult to explain. I don't know. I feel that it's one thing caring for somebody who's sick. Helping them to get better or even helping them towards a good death, that makes sense but I have never been to see myself as a midwife.'

'Is that really how you see it?'

'Yes. I'm sorry: I don't want to do it. I don't think I have a calling for it. I have prayed and prayed, and the same answer comes back: I can't face a future like that.'

I was stunned. Cecilia had been my role model. We sat in silence for some minutes and then she changed the subject.

'And then there's Sister Julia.'

I nodded. Cecilia and I weren't the only ones to be moved around. In fact there seemed to be a policy of moving all of us, every few years. It was probably something to do with not wanting us to become too settled, a need to feel they were challenging us. Sister Julia had been offered the job of midwife tutor at the hospital two years before and as her pupils, we were going to have to see her every day, be examined by her and in fact were dependent on her assessment of us in order to be able to pass. Cecilia had never had an easy relationship with Sister Julia and that added to her difficulties.

'I begged to be allowed to go to King's College Hospital but Mother wasn't having any of it.'

'Did you? Gosh, Cecilia, good for you! What did she say?'

'She said it would look most irregular to send one of the Community to be trained somewhere else when one of the Sisters is the midwife tutor at the Lying-In Hospital.'

'Well, perhaps she has a point?'

'Nonsense! It shouldn't be about what things look like and anyway who's going to notice, and as you well know, we have a long connection with King's.'

That was true. The first school of midwifery was set up by the Community of St John's at King's College Hospital.

Cecilia's tone then became more sad and serious. 'I don't know why I'm being tested now. Why, when I have just committed myself for life? It's too late.'

'Perhaps that's why. You're being tested because it's safe.'

Cecilia looked unconvinced. I was unconvinced. My words sounded a bit trite, and the thought crept into my mind that perhaps it wasn't so much God choosing this moment to test Cecilia; but that she was indeed right, this was not her calling.

However, this was the only time that Cecilia and I spoke about her feelings about midwifery and her vocation. This was something that I was later to sorely regret; but as the weeks went on, although I could tell she wasn't fully engaged, she seemed to be settling in, and I took her at face value. It wasn't just in the religious life that discussion of problems was difficult, but the whole of British society still had its imperial stiff upper lip in place. Although I prided myself on not being taken in by the system, I guess this was one of the signs that despite my best efforts, I had become part of it.

Cecilia's doubts were also pushed out of my head because from the day I started, I loved training to be a midwife. The General Lying-In Hospital was opposite St Thomas's Hospital on the South Bank in central London. It looked out onto the Thames and the Houses of Parliament, which felt pretty exciting after five years in Hastings. Since I had been away, London had climbed out of its dreary post-war austerity and was just starting to swing. Even a Sister could appreciate the excitement of the new freedom of the young – the clothes, the music, the relaxation in formality. Even if I couldn't fully participate, I felt as if the mood would somehow percolate down to me.

The work itself was exciting and absorbing. Most of our training took place on the wards, with a weekly study day. It was organised so that we each spent some time in every area of the maternity hospital – the antenatal clinic, the antenatal ward, the labour ward, the post-natal ward and the special care baby nursery. In this way it was easy to link what we learned in the classroom to what we saw and experienced on the wards. What I found especially useful was the requirement that every time we witnessed a baby's delivery, we were sent to interview the mother a couple of days later. We asked them what was helpful, what could have been done better? Of course I had my own impression about how it had all gone, but the mother's perspective was often quite different. It gave me all sorts of insights that helped when I started to be in charge of deliveries myself.

Unlike today, where mothers seem to be discharged as soon as possible, in the Sixties mothers were expected to spend the first ten days after giving birth in hospital, basically resting. Yes, they were encouraged to get up and have a walk around, but the main purpose of their stay was to make sure they recovered and healed. It worries me that today too much is expected of a new mother; it seems to have been forgotten, or perhaps ignored for financial reasons, how exhausting giving birth is. It's vital that a woman is feeling as well and as strong as possible when she starts out on those first crucial, intense and exhausting months of her baby's life.

Keeping new mothers in hospital meant that we carried on building our relationships with them, which in turn meant we were better able to help mothers settle, bond, and feed their babies, and pick up potential problems. We helped them to give their babies their first bath, change them and get them into a routine. Every night we tucked the mothers up and took the babies into the nursery so the mothers slept. Generally the babies, first fed then carefully swaddled in the dimly lit nursery, slept too. We fed them, or took them to their mothers to be fed, every three or four hours to start getting them into some sort of a routine. Generally this was very successful and it felt like we were establishing them and getting them off to a good start.

When the mothers went home from hospital their care was taken over by the community midwives and then the health visitors. The downside of building up these relationships is that when the mothers left the hospital you didn't know what happened to them. I remember working in the post-natal ward and meeting a 14-year-old girl who had just given birth to her first baby, a little girl. In between looking after her baby, she would read *Jane Eyre*. I wanted to weep for her. I don't know what happened to her. Perhaps her baby was given up for adoption, but whatever did happen, her life had been changed forever. But then I also learned not to jump to conclusions. A young woman was rushed in to deliver twins early, at 30 weeks of pregnancy. She already had one set of twins who were only 18 months old. One afternoon I was in the special care unit and she was standing between the two incubators where her twins were lying and holding each of their hands.

'Aren't I lucky?' she said. 'They're all mine.'

I couldn't stop the thought going through my head that if it was me, I'd hand one set back but she was obviously seeing things a bit differently. I was left wondering what would become of some of these mothers and babies. It seemed perilous sending some of them back out to face the tough city beyond.

But of course the most critical part of our training was in the labour ward. The first time I witnessed a birth was the most extraordinary experience. The bell rang and I dashed off to the delivery room, feeling that I was probably as excited (and nervous) as the mother. It was a routine delivery of a young 20-year-old having her first baby. As was usual in those days, the father wasn't present. The mother was in the final stages. We may have been in a modern, bright hospital room but there was something essentially primeval going on. The midwife, however, was calm and concentrating, talking her through. The mother's sheer phenomenal effort and energy filled the room and it was difficult to witness. I felt my body wanting to push too, to help: I felt like she needed it. However, despite the initial appearance to the contrary, no help was needed; a head appeared and then another phenomenal push and the baby was born.

It was one of the most moving things I had ever seen. Of course at one level I knew a baby was going to come out, but it wasn't until I had seen him emerge that it really hit me. A baby, a real live baby, another human life had entered the world! It didn't seem possible and yet I had witnessed it myself, with my very own eyes.

As I watched the mother hold her new baby son in her arms, silently gazing at him, a sudden picture of calm and peace after the tremendous struggle, I was struck by the feeling that no birth could ever be commonplace and that feeling has never left me. I don't know how anyone could see a baby being born and not be moved to the very core of their being. It's a sacred time, the miracle of life playing out in front of your eyes. This was my first overwhelming impression. But during my training a slower realisation dawned: it became apparent that getting to know each mother was very important, so as to be able to support her at this vital time in her life.

The general rule was that we had to witness about five deliveries before we were gradually allowed to start delivering ourselves. I say 'gradually' because at first you would be delivering, but with the midwife's hands on top of your own. It's one thing to be in a classroom practising with a doll going through a plastic pelvis, quite another to be there in the heat of the action, down at the business end.

It was at this point that I was really struck with how much midwifery is an art as well as a science. The midwife intuitively seemed to know exactly the right place to put her hands, exactly the right amount of pressure to put on the baby. Her hands felt so alive and flexible, totally responding to the smallest changes in movement and pressure. She explained how critical it was to know exactly which position the baby was in while trying to enter the world. Through finding the angle of the sutures and fontanelles she would know whether the baby was coming in an anterior or posterior position (basically, facing the front or facing the back) and from the size of the birth canal and the head whether the baby would be able to come out without assistance, or whether a cut would have to be made or, indeed, whether the mother would need a Caesarean.

As the labour reached the final stages the midwife would place the pad of her left hand at the mother's rectum and her right hand would feel the baby's head, constantly checking the bones and the position of the suture lines, which are where the bony plates of the baby's skull meet, and the fontanelles, the soft spots in the plates which are flexible during birth to allow the baby's head to squeeze down the birth canal. I very quickly had a sense when a delivery had gone well, and this was not only when both mother and baby came out of the experience healthy and intact, but also when a mother had felt that she herself had enabled her child to come into the world.

Of course there were times when this was not possible. In the Sixties in London it was normal for a first-time mother to have her baby in hospital. However, as long as there were no complications, subsequent babies were often born at home. This meant that in the hospital we saw more high-risk cases and there were far more complications than if we were working on the district.

One day a woman came in with very strange amniocentesis results. I was worried when I met her in the antenatal clinic. It wasn't possible from the results to actually pin down what might be wrong with the baby; they were strange in the most unusual way. It seemed impossible to believe that the baby could be normal and healthy. Of course there was just the possibility that this was a rogue test but I couldn't seem to shift the alarm bells in my head. Obviously the doctors thought so too, because they insisted that she give birth in hospital. And when summoned by the bell, I rushed into the delivery room to see this lady in the final stages of labour. I was filled with foreboding. It wasn't just the medical warnings; I think it is possible to have a sixth sense about these things. As the baby emerged, I saw the horrified look on the midwife's face and then she did something I've never seen before – she turned away.

'Catherine, can you get the consultant for me?'

The midwife in charge was very experienced and her voice was calm, but her face had gone grey. I walked purposefully out of the room and then ran down the corridor. Luckily, the obstetrician was on his rounds and easy to track down. We hurried back into the room. By this time the baby had just come out. I caught one glimpse of him; that's all I needed. Where there should have been eyes, there were none. Instead he had one large eye in the middle of his forehead. He was a cyclopia, commonly known as a Cyclops baby.

It's a very rare condition, usually caused by the mother being exposed to toxins in early pregnancy. The baby's eyes do not develop and a large eye in the centre of the forehead appears instead. Often the baby's other organs have not developed normally either. Usually a Cyclops baby will live for only a few hours. I have to say that one brief glimpse of the poor child has seared itself into my memory. One of my first instincts was to pick him up and comfort him. I was attracted and yet deeply repelled; I couldn't bring myself to be the one to step forward and pick him up. One of the nurses did clean him, wrap him up and take him out of the room. After that I don't know where he was taken or what happened to him for sure, but I believe that he did die after a couple of hours, as these babies have no chance of survival for any length of time with this extreme disability.

I was left in the room with his mother and the staff midwife. The mother was not told what was wrong with him, but she was told that her child had a gross abnormality and sadly, would not live, and that the doctor would come and see her shortly. We did our best to comfort her in this distressing situation where everyone present was upset.

Later that night when I got back, relieved to be in the peace and safety of my little room, I prayed for a long time. I had been shocked at my own inability to help the poor baby. My courage had failed when it was most needed. I felt terribly guilty; I also wondered whether the baby had had a chance to be baptised. I prayed:

'Please God, forgive me. I'm so sorry. Poor, poor child. I'm sorry I couldn't comfort this baby. When You needed me to act, I failed. I am so sorry, forgive me, Lord. I wasn't there for your child.'

But whatever doubts I had became totally insignificant when I finally got to deliver my first baby all by myself. For the second part of my training I had to spend six months working with the Community delivering babies at home. It felt so right to be back in Poplar, like coming full circle in a good way. When I walked into the old square with the huge All Saints church on one side, then at right angles to it the big house where I had lived in my late teens and had so many happy times as a parish worker, and going on to live in the big Mission House on the third side of the square, it felt very satisfactory. I had come back, but in a new incarnation – in a Sister's habit, as if fulfilling the prophecy that had first been revealed to me in Old Sue's flat, just around the corner.

I had been back once before, in my first year in the convent. I was invited to the wedding of one of my fellow parish worker's and the handsome young curate who had taken a fancy to my hat. I'd taken the invitation to Mother Sarah Grace, who'd stared at it for a long time as if trying to read between the lines.

'You can go back, but only to the service. You must come home before the reception.'

And before I knew it, that question had popped out again.

'But why, Mother?'

'You might miss the last train.'

'But it starts very early, I'm sure I could pop in for just an hour.'

There was a moment of silence and then I could see resistance was futile.

'Yes, Mother,' I said quickly.

I withdrew from the study immediately, feeling like a holy Cinderella: condemned to receive an invitation but never to go to the ball. Strangely enough the day before the wedding, Mother Sarah Grace stopped me in the cloister and said, 'Catherine Mary, you may go to the reception, but you must be sure you are on the last train home.'

I have no idea what changed her mind, but I still felt like Cinderella. Now the fairy godmother had given me permission to go as long as I was back by midnight (except that Jesus was my prince and I had sensible shoes instead of glass slippers).

My first impression was that Poplar, a bit like myself, was the same and yet fundamentally different. It was a world that was changing very fast. A bit like the modern-day city of Rome, the old layers were there and could still be seen poking through, but new layers were being built on top very fast. While there was still rubble left on the bomb sites from the Blitz, half the old tenement buildings had been taken down, new buildings were going up and some shiny high-rise blocks towered above the whole scene. But many of the same old faces and families that I had known from five years earlier were still there; it still felt like a second home.

It was an interesting and dynamic time to be working on the district; we all had to learn fast. My tutor was Sister Alice. Again, she had a firm manner. However, I experienced her differently to Sister Julia because underneath, I found her rather soft. I realised this quite early on: I had only been there a couple of weeks and it was Ash Wednesday (indeed, the fifth anniversary of my arrival in the religious life) when I'd been out all night following the duty midwife at two difficult deliveries and by the time I'd unpacked my bag and sterilised my equipment, I felt totally washed out. I knew I had just three hours to get some kind of sleep before I must attend the afternoon antenatal clinic. As I climbed wearily and somewhat despondently up the stairs to my room, Sister Alice came round the corner and glided down the stairs, beckoning me towards her.

'Give me your hand,' she demanded.

Rather scared, I did as I was told. From inside the folds of her habit she produced a small, bulging, white paper bag and pressed it into my hand.

'For you,' she said. 'For Lent.' And she moved swiftly on down the stairs.

When I got to my room I opened the bag. Inside were exactly 40 large mint humbugs: one for every day in Lent. I was so touched. I ate one a day for the next 40 days and with each one, I felt a wave of love for my tutor. After that I couldn't see her without a metaphorical golden halo above the top of her head, no matter how stern her manner.

I spent the first three months dutifully working with the midwife and gradually I was allowed to do more. Finally, one day I was called out to attend what was expected to be a routine birth. I arrived at 7 p.m. By 7.30 the mother was in the final stages of labour and I knew the midwife was not going to be there in time, but I felt totally calm and ready. A few minutes later I delivered a healthy baby boy; the mother called him John.

I was overjoyed. It was my 25th birthday and it seemed wholly appropriate he should be called the name of our patron saint.

CHAPTER SIX

THE EMPTY PLACE

It all started with an empty place at the dinner table at the Mission House. Usually we all ate lunch together at a large wooden square table in a room rather grandly referred to as the 'refectory' even though it would have been a bit poky as a dining room in a country vicarage. The unspoken rule was that we all sat in the same places; there was quiet consternation and a gentle whispered correction when an unsuspecting visitor happened to sit in one of our seats. In line with tradition at the Mother House, the head of the House, Sister Ruth, sat at the top of the table, while the Sisters sat down from her according to their unofficial place in the hierarchy. So next came my tutor, Sister Alice, and the Sister I'd brought to Old Sue, Sister Dorothy, then Sisters Belinda and Sarah Jane, followed by Cecilia and me sitting opposite each other with the five trainee nurse midwives down at the bottom end.

Today Sister Cecilia wasn't there. Normally Sister Ruth would wait until everyone was present and standing behind their chairs before she said grace. Today she said grace even though there was no Cecilia. I thought it was slightly odd. Turning to Sister Belinda, I asked, 'Has there been an emergency?'

I noticed she looked a bit on edge and she couldn't look me in the eye.

'No.'

'I was just wondering where Sister Cecilia might be.'

Looks passed between Sisters Ruth, Alice and Dorothy. There was silence and they bent over their plates and carried on eating. I got the message: I was obviously not supposed to know, or at least be asking.

I was busy in the clinic in the afternoon, but when we went into our little chapel for Evening Prayer and Cecilia wasn't in her usual place in the pew, I knew something was wrong. Then I felt even more anxious when there was still an empty place at supper. As soon as I'd finished my meal, I headed up to the top floor where the Sisters had their bedrooms. All the rooms in the Mission House had been given names, typed in large letters and pinned to the doors. Some of them didn't seem entirely appropriate – the office was called 'Love', the patients' waiting room 'Wisdom', the kitchen 'Counsel' and I had the honour of a small bedroom on the top floor called 'Endurance'. Cecilia's bedroom was the last one at the end of the corridor and called 'The Prophet's Chamber'.

I knocked on the door. There was no sound. I tentatively pushed it open. There was nothing. No Cecilia, and none of her things; only clean, neatly folded sheets on the bed and a clear desk. Her pictures of the Virgin and the Crucifixion were gone from the walls. I opened the wardrobe but there was just a rail of empty coat hangers. Then I wondered whether I had got the right room. I backed out and looked at the name on the door. Yes, 'The Prophet's Chamber'.

I felt like I was going mad. I headed straight for Sister Ruth's office, but walking was difficult; I had run out of air. I dreaded what I was about to hear, but then I knew I wouldn't be able to shake this feeling until I'd asked the question. She couldn't have gone. Maybe she's ill, I thought, and with horror I realised that would actually feel like good news.

The worst news would be that Cecilia had gone. But leaving after she had taken her life vows would be very unusual. Many women realise that the religious life is not for them in the early stages – perhaps only a tenth of those who start on the journey end up taking their life vows. But once they have been through all those years of testing, very few ever leave. In my whole time at the Community, none of the Sisters had gone – not least because it is very difficult to revoke lifetime vows.

Of course it is possible to just walk out of the door but most women who leave don't do that. You have to imagine what you might feel after living so many years in Community. You have, effectively, consecrated yourself to the service of Christ. It would be like walking out on a marriage without ever getting divorced – unfinished business and impossible to marry someone else unless bigamy was your thing. So to be officially released from your vows, you have to undergo another long process of examination. Cecilia would first have had to apply to Sister Ruth and then she would have had to stand in front of a special Chapter of the Sisters, where they would listen very carefully to what she had to say and give their advice. After prayerful discussion, a period of what is rather sinisterly known as 'exclaustration' is generally (although not always) offered. This is a specified cooling-off period, where a Sister would be allowed to leave and live outside the Community. It usually lasts two or three years and is a difficult time. She would be given a small allowance by the Community but effectively she would be on her own. Often Sisters would choose to go home to their parents, but I knew Cecilia's parents were both dead. Where would she go? And even then, at the end of this period, if she still wished to be released from her vows, a letter from the Bishop would have to be sent to the Archbishop of Canterbury, asking him for secularisation.

I tried to imagine Cecilia going through this long ordeal on her own. Leaving was seen as an act of disloyalty, a failure. The prospect of facing such a long intense process filled me with dread.

Feeling sick, I knocked on the door to Sister Ruth's office. It was marked 'Hope'. I couldn't help it, but every time I knocked on it, the words went through my head,

'Abandon it all ye who enter here', and today was no different. I had the feeling I was about to step over one of those lines and do something stupid.

Sister Ruth was tiny and inscrutable. Though generally an approachable and kind lady, 'communication issues' was a phrase we quietly muttered to each other. She could make anything a secret. Rumour had it that before she became a Sister, she used to work for the Intelligence Services. On reflection, there are many skills that are transferable between being a spy and being a Sister – obedience to orders, total discretion and impenetrability, to mention but a few.

I walked in. Sister Ruth looked pale but then she always looked pale. It had constantly amazed me how most of the Sisters had eventually managed to perfect inscrutable faces: Sister Ruth was a master at it. I looked to see any sign of worry. There was the usual blank canvas.

'And how might I help you, Sister Catherine Mary?'

'It's Sister Cecilia. I don't understand. She's not been here all day. I've just been to her room; it's completely clear of all her things.'

'Indeed.'

'So you know?'

'Yes.'

There was silence. I couldn't believe it. That was all she was going to say. I could feel red-hot anger starting to bubble up from the depths.

'Has she gone to the Mother House?'

'No.'

'Well, where is she?'

'It is not for you to know.'

'Not for me to *know*?'

There was a pause. That was really all she was going to say.

'Not for me to *know*? Not for me to *know*? I don't believe you! My friend has disappeared and it's not for me to know!'

'I beg your pardon, Sister Catherine Mary. Collect yourself at once. You have lost control. It does not befit you or any member of our Community.'

'You call this a Community? Someone can just disappear off the face of the earth and no one will talk about it? As if she never existed? I mean, is she ill, is she alright?'

There was more silence.

'Don't you care?'

Sister Ruth took a deep breath and seemed to slightly soften.

'Sister Cecilia has decided to leave us and I doubt whether you will ever see her again. I think you need to go and spend time praying for her and her future.'

I hovered uncertainly; I didn't want to leave Cecilia's fate so unresolved. I had no idea where this rage was coming from. It didn't feel like me; I didn't even know I had it in me. In the end there was a sensible voice talking quietly but firmly over the rage, telling me to just pause and think before I crossed a line I probably wouldn't be able to come back from, so I just turned my back and left.

I sat in my room – 'Endurance' – in the dark, wracking my brains trying to work out just what had happened. Cecilia had gone, but where? Forever? Just like that, without telling me. It didn't seem possible that someone could just disappear. I couldn't accept it, not without being given some kind of reason. And why hadn't I known? Why hadn't she talked to me? I felt rage at the stupidity and inhumanity of the Sisters, but also rage towards Cecilia, leaving me here like this. I tried to imagine a world without her and her friendship, and it was horrible. I felt abandoned in a cold empty universe, spinning alone. And then I wondered whether it was actually me who had abandoned her. I remembered the conversation on our first night at the hospital. I didn't know for certain but my instincts were telling me that I already knew why she had gone: she didn't want to be a midwife, she must have been suffering all this time and I hadn't noticed. But then why hadn't she talked to me? Why on earth had they made her carry on if she was finding it so difficult? There was plenty of demand for plain district nursing in the parish. And then the big question: if she had gone, why was I still here?

I prayed: 'Dear God, forgive me. I'm supposed to be a Christian. I've devoted my life to the service of others and yet I missed the need of my best friend right here under my nose.'

I went on, 'Dear God, forgive me my anger towards the Sisters and towards Cecilia too.'

And I lay on my bed in my habit and spent the whole night awake with my mind racing on its own hellish motorway of 'if onlys', speeding up as the dark receded and the morning light started to come in through the window.

As the bell to rise began to ring, I got up and automatically went through my morning routine. I joined the Sisters wending their way across the square in their black capes to the parish church of All Saints for our early-morning Communion. The church was right in the middle of the square; a large, beautiful mid nineteenth-century church built in a classical style, with steps up to a grand entrance flanked by large columns. Inside was uncluttered. There were no stained-glass windows, only clear glass, giving a sense of space and light, room for the spirit to roam free, space to think. There were two side chapels, one with a beautiful statue of Our Lady, but the small chapel of the Blessed Sacrament was where we usually had our early-morning communion.

This church and I were old friends. I had spent many hours in there as a parish worker. Sometimes I felt as if I could almost catch a glimpse of my younger un-nunned self sitting in her seat in the main church in the middle of the left aisle. This idea had always given me comfort. I was on a journey, making a natural progression through the church as I went up the ladder towards God – the same person in the same church and yet transformed and about to be transformed again. Today this thought brought me no comfort. In fact, I had no sense of it at all. Instead I wanted to grab my younger self and say 'Run!'. Usually I felt held and comforted by my silent older Sister companions, one of a Community. Today, the black capes either side of me felt oppressive. Now that one of us had escaped, I felt imprisoned. I tried to pray but my lines of communication with the Divine were silent. 'Is there anyone out there at all?' was the question that popped into my head.

As we walked back, we were usually hit by the smell of freshly baked bread coming from the cellar of the bakery on the square. I was always hungry by this time (often I felt as if I were about to faint at the altar rail as I took Communion) and the smell of the bread tipped me over into a ravenous frenzy. Today, it made me feel sick. When I tried to eat my breakfast, my buttered toast tasted like cardboard: one bite and it stuck in my throat. My cup of tea was good, though. It's amazing how tea never fails to hit the spot in emotional crises. I noticed there was no longer an empty place in front of me; the nurses had all moved up one.

For the next couple of days I struggled with work. One afternoon I was in the antenatal clinic. In a way it was easier just to go through the motions in the clinic. There was a bit of a routine: we'd ask the mother how she had been since her last visit, we'd weigh her and take her blood pressure, put her on the bed and measure the baby, and make a note of its lie and presentation. We'd ask how she was eating and, if her pregnancy was well advanced, we would make sure she was making all the right preparations. I was doing all the right things, but I wasn't really concentrating. I kept asking questions and then missing the answers and having to ask my mothers to repeat them. When I asked one lady for the third time whether she was all right, she replied, 'I'm all right, Sister, are you all right?'

I also had to check the mother's urine to make sure that there was no protein present. In those days we had to boil the urine in a test tube over a Bunsen burner. I was standing holding the test tube in the flame, obviously away with the fairies, because suddenly there was a crack and the glass shattered. Shards of glass and hot urine splashed my habit and flew across the room.

I noticed it wasn't only me who was suffering. Before she entered the religious life, Sister Belinda had been a concert pianist. She was now a quiet devout woman, probably in her late fifties. Although we had an old upright piano in the Community Room, 'Charity', we were not allowed to play it. That evening, as I walked past the door, I saw Sister Belinda go up to the piano and kick it. I worked out that it was probably 30 years since she had last been allowed to play a piano.

I urgently needed to talk to someone about Cecilia, but with no Cecilia, there was no one to talk to. When I found myself alone with Sister Dorothy that evening, her face bent low over her needlework, I took a risk and said, 'Sister Dorothy, I wonder do you know what happened to Sister Cecilia?'

She didn't lift her head but carried on sewing and said with a snort, 'Silly girl! Fancy giving up all this.'

I looked round the room, 'Charity', and for the first time imagined what it must look like to an outsider. Two Sisters, one older, one younger, sitting in the semi-darkness, crouched over needlework. A dusty piano that never got played, a couple of old standard lamps with heavy, mismatched floral shades, ten stiff-back armchairs arranged round the edge of the room with, again, various floral coverings, some more worn than others, a dark brown carpet and a rather sorry-looking aspidistra plant. I nearly laughed.

Officially of course there was someone we could talk to. Once a month we had to go and confess our sins to our chaplain. Father Matthew was an ageing member of the Anglican Society of St John the Evangelist, otherwise known as the Cowley Fathers. They were strict with a tradition of 'custody of the eyes'. This meant they were careful about making eye contact so that, as much as possible, they avoided images that could lead to sinful thoughts. I remember being affronted one day when travelling back from a visit to the Mother House in Hastings. I walked into a carriage and Father Matthew was already sitting down. I sat opposite him, all ready to make polite conversation, but he totally refused to acknowledge me and we spent the whole hour and a half-long journey in silence, not looking at each other! For the last five years I'd been pouring out my official innermost darkest secrets to him and he couldn't even acknowledge me in a train carriage. Of course by avoiding making eye contact with me Father Matthew was just fulfilling the requirements of his Order, but it was this kind of institutionalised rigidity that got on my nerves. Would Christ have done that?

Of course I hadn't really been pouring out my innermost thoughts to him. Along with most of the Sisters, I think, I presented him with a made-up list of things I hadn't done. As he appeared brusque and really the last person you would actually want to confide in, the whole exercise seemed a little pointless. My real confessions went straight in prayer to God. However, at this point I decided to give him one last chance.

Confession took place in the sacristy of the small chapel in Deptford. At my allotted time I walked down the dark stairs to the little crypt lit by candles underneath. Father Matthew sat on his chair, facing away from me. I knelt at the small bench called the prie-dieu and stared at the crucifix on the wall. Father Matthew was dressed in his plain black habit, tied round the middle with a rope with its three knots and a crucifix hanging from it. He was still facing in the opposite direction. As I have said, eye contact was something to be avoided. The whole exercise was terribly formal. I started with the prescribed words, 'Bless me, Father, for I have sinned …'

I then said the standard Prayer of Penitence. The Confession was a bit more tricky and you had to put some thought into it. It always had to be about the negative, having difficulty with meditation, being so busy with work that we forgot to say our offices, the difficult relations with a certain Sister. It was like a shopping list of minor sins. Today, I was determined to make it more meaningful.

'Sister Catherine Mary, may you speak with honesty before your God, what have you to tell me?'

Determined for once to actually speak the truth, I concentrated on the crucifix and started to speak.

'Father, I am struggling. Deeply struggling. Sister Cecilia has left and I am finding it difficult. I don't understand why she has gone. No one will tell me and I am feeling angry: angry that she has left without speaking to me, angry towards the Sisters for not seeming to care. I am left wondering who she was, who the Sisters are. Everything looks different and most of all, I miss her …'

He stopped me in my tracks.

'Sister Catherine Mary, get a hold of yourself! What are you saying?'

I struggled to keep back the tears.

'Father, please listen to me. I don't think I can go on.'

'Well, Sister you've got to deal with it! Give it up to God … Immediately.'

At this point I looked round at his back, willing him to turn round. He did not stir.

'Give it up to God, Catherine Mary, give it up.'

I took a deep breath and stopped. I could not say another word. He said a quick prayer of Absolution, gave me a penance of prayers and I left. I didn't look at him again.

The next day I was on my way to deliver a baby when my bicycle wheel hit a patch of ice and I came tumbling off and hit my head on the kerb.

'All right, Sister?' a man dropped his workbag and picked me up.

'Yes, yes, I think so, thanks,' I said as I smoothed down my habit.

'Are you sure, love? You didn't 'arf 'it your 'ead 'ard.'

'I'm fine, thank you very much.'

'Well, look after yourself, treacle.'

'Um … thanks.'

Treacle? I had an image of gooey sticky liquid penetrating my brain as I wobbled off down the road. The delivery was, thankfully, straightforward. It was a third child for a laid-back, salt-of-the-earth Cockney woman. Within the hour a new baby boy had arrived in the world but as I leant over the bath to examine the dish that held the placenta, I suddenly felt a terrible throbbing in my head and then I blacked out. The next thing I knew, I was lying on the bed with a newborn baby in the cot beside me.

''Ere, love, 'ave a cuppa. You 'ad a nasty turn.'

The poor mother, who'd only given birth half an hour ago, was standing over me with a cup of tea. At this moment Sister Alice, having completed her routine rounds, walked into the room. The look on her face when she saw me lying in bed with a newborn baby beside me was priceless.

That evening, after all the prayers, I was sitting in my room staring into space, still with a slight headache, when there was gentle knock on the door. It was Sister Alice. She came into the room and sat on my bed.

'Sister dear, you are sad. Something is not right.'

'Yes, Sister Alice.'

'I was wondering if I could help.'

Sister Alice was my midwifery tutor and it was not her job to look after my pastoral care, so with that first piece of humanity and evidence of love, I started to cry. When I used to cry when I was little, my mother would say, 'Just look at those crocodile tears! I've never seen any so big,' and she and my siblings would laugh at me, which didn't really help. Sister Alice was more sympathetic and drew me to her impressive bosom and gave me a hug. I hadn't been hugged for six years. In the 1960s Sisters were discouraged from anything other than the most minimal greeting peck on the cheek. The wonder of human physical contact. I had so missed it, and I blurted out randomly a whole host of things I had been holding inside.

'I am so confused, so lonely. I've lost my way. Everything looks different; I don't know where I am. I thought I knew, but now I don't. I don't know anyone any more.'

'You feel lost at the moment, don't you?'

'Yes, yes, I do. I don't know how to find my way out.'

I had to stop speaking while I cried some more, big childish sobs. Sister Alice's habit was getting wet.

'You have lost the path.'

'Yes, and I'm so scared.'

My nose was running and dripping onto her habit. She couldn't see. My head was on her shoulder.

'It's Cecilia. I can't seem to get past her going. I don't understand it. I don't understand how it could have happened. Why didn't she speak to me? I miss her so much. But I can't make sense of it. No one will talk to me about it; it's like she's been erased. But she hasn't: not in my heart.'

I had pulled back from her shoulder and I was jabbing at my chest, and I could hear with some alarm that my voice was raised.

'You're angry.'

'Yes. Yes. I'm really, really angry. Angry with her, angry with me … angry with all of you, just going along as if nothing has happened. As if she doesn't matter.'

Sister Alice remained calm. There was silence as we both listened to the echo of my words and then she asked, 'And angry with God?'

'Yes. Yes, OK then, yes. I'm angry with God.'

'And what is He telling you?'

'Nothing, absolutely nothing.'

'You have prayed?'

'Oh Sister, of course I've jolly well prayed. But He isn't listening.'

There was a shocked silence, or rather my shocked silence. She didn't seem to notice, or perhaps chose not to notice, that I was actually shouting at her now.

'You have told Him that you are angry with Him?'

I paused. I thought about it and said a bit more quietly, 'No. No, I suppose I haven't. But I can't hear or feel Him. It's like He just vanished in Cecilia's suitcase.'

'Perhaps you are just too angry to let Him in. Because He is here, you know. He hasn't gone. Perhaps it is you that has gone off in Cecilia's suitcase.'

She was smiling at me now. I couldn't help but smile back through the tears. I loved her calm certainty, it was very reassuring, and holding and infectious.

'Catherine Mary, you have to be real with God. You have to take your anger to Him. You have to sit with Him, tell Him you are angry with Him and tell Him why. Use your tears; make them your prayer. In order to grow in love with God you have to be real, you have to present all shades of your being to Him, even the angry ones.'

She paused, drew a hanky from the folds of her habit and wiped away my tears. I felt like a child.

'Sometimes God is absent. That is when we most need our faith and patience. He will come back if we let

Him and are truly open to Him. As you know sometimes He doesn't speak to us directly but wherever you look, there are references to Him. He shows Himself through other people, small acts of kindness. I saw Him at work this afternoon when you were lying on the bed with the miracle of life beside you and a new mother had got up and made you a cup of tea. Once I had got over my surprise, I felt deeply moved. It was a beautiful nativity scene and put me in mind of Jesus's unlikely start in a manger and the innkeeper's grace.'

I pictured what Sister Alice had seen. I hadn't thought about it like that at all. Well, I wasn't really thinking – I had a really throbbing headache – but suddenly I felt moved too.

'Sister Alice, could you tell me about what happened to Cecilia? Just a little. Just something that might help me to understand.'

'Of course it's against our rules to discuss these matters, but yes, I am moved to tell you. Perhaps it is the Holy Spirit reaching out to you, Catherine. Sometimes we are called to break earthly rules by something higher. Anyway, Sister Cecilia did not want to be a midwife. She did not believe this was her calling and this brought into question her whole calling to the religious life. She has gone away to consider these questions. What concerns me at this moment is that it seems to have had an impact on your calling.'

'Yes, it's like my foundation has been pulled away. I suddenly feel as if I'm the house built on sand rather than on stone.'

'But is it sand? You see, I've always felt your calling to this work, to being a midwife, is very, very solid. To walk with someone in childbirth, coping with their pain and suffering, to seek and find God in the context of bringing new life into the world, I witness you feeling this, in a way that Cecilia never did.'

An image came to mind of my first baby, little John.

'Yes, Sister, I have felt that.'

'Then you are in the right place, doing the right thing. If the work and the life brings you closer to God, if you feel God beside you when you do this, you are in the right place; you are called.'

I nodded. Sister Alice had given me a glimpse of the path again.

'But I do think you need a rest and some space to be with God. There is some need for an opportunity for reconciliation. I want you to take a couple of days off – stay in your room, go for walks, it doesn't matter – but I would like you to attend prayers. In the meantime I want to give you this.'

From inside the folds of her habit she produced a small, worn leather notebook.

'I would like to read the diary of one of our Community who was also called and managed to find God in the most extreme situation. Read, be with Nurse Wren, and God and pray. You will find a way back. Your calling is built on the most solid foundations. It is built on stone, I know that, my child.'

Sister Alice left and for the first time since Sister Cecilia had disappeared, I experienced some kind of peace and slept soundly.

The next morning I woke up early and started turning the fragile pages of Nurse Wren's diary. Out slipped an old sepia photograph of a lady standing in what looked like a muddy farmyard. She had big gumboots on her feet, a long sensible overcoat with an ethnic satchel strapped across her body, and a floppy felt hat. Her head was tipped slightly quizzically to one side and she had a determined yet kind expression. I thought that perhaps she was only in her mid-twenties. I started to read her words and was immediately plunged into the chaos of the First World War. On the first page Nurse Wren wrote,

> *It was pitiful to see quite tiny children with both feet and often one hand swollen and discoloured, absolutely helpless to treat apart from amputation, which they dread most of all.*

I realised straight away that this was not going to be an easy read.

Nurse Wren had been working for the Community of St John when in August 1915 she was sent to help care for the casualties of the fighting in Serbia. At first she appeared to be in good spirits and described a chaotic journey on a jolting bullock wagon, being thrown on to the laps of the good women of the Scottish missionary hospital to the amusement of the local townsfolk. But on arriving in camp she was faced with a typhoid epidemic.

We were badly needed in camp as many of the staff were slowly recovering from typhoid fever and the number of patients were daily increasing ... often they came two and three days journey by bullock wagon as there are few doctors left in Serbia since the typhus scurge. Tuberculosis is rife, as is cancer.

Nurse Wren set to work with good humour, cheerily describing nights spent battling with tents, ropes and pegs as she tried to cope with the vicious Balkan storms,

Quite amusing, only being unused to the ropes, one had a fair amount of tumbles! I fear few of our English acquaintances would scarcely have recognized us when we came off duty in the mornings.

She had only been there a month when the Germans started to bomb the camp. As bombs dropped around it seemed their only protection was to close the tent flaps. It soon became obvious more effective measures were needed and the patients were moved a few miles and ended up strewn along the roadsides in all sorts of strange garments. But the Germans were advancing quickly. They were given orders to discharge all the civil patients.

That was very sad, so many were quite unfit to travel. Bullock wagons were commandeered by the government and trains were no longer available, these days are not easy to write about.

As the Germans began to bombard Belgrade the casualties started to pour in.

Their wounds were fearful and we wondered how they managed to get to us, some had been five days without any attention and little food.

More than half could not be admitted. They had run out of beds and food, and many were just left by the roadside.

The Serbs slept with their blankets pulled over their heads so every night Nurse Wren had to go round checking they had not died. It was particularly important as, according to Serbian tradition, they should have been holding a lit candle in their hands as they passed into the shadows. Her night shifts were spent trying to make sure this happened.

As Belgrade fell they made preparations to leave camp. With no food, Nurse Wren said the discomfort of the patients was 'indescribable'. However, she said that they did not complain and did not fear death, and put their trust in the medical staff. Then, on 25 October, they were given the order to march and they had to leave their patients behind to the mercy of the Enemy. She described it as heart-rending but 'our training imposes strict obedience. I dare not judge.' Ah yes, the 'O' word. I could identify with that.

I decided to put on my black cape and go for a walk. Outside, Poplar was busy. It was a spring day, with breezy fluffy clouds and bright sunshine across a light blue sky; clear and contrasting with the hectic, messy world underneath. There was building work everywhere. On the ruined bomb sites there were cranes constructing new tower blocks. The streets were filled with busy, optimistic women in headscarves with shopping bags and men with cigarettes in their mouths, looking purposeful. Children were crowding the streets on their way home from school. The war had been over for nearly 20 years, life was renewing itself, the world was moving on; but was it moving on without me?

I didn't feel able to go back to the diary until the evening. What then unfolded was the story of Nurse Wren and her party's dramatic hike across a snow-covered Serbia, chased by the rapidly advancing German Army. The aim was to get to the coast to catch a boat out of the war zone. I was struck by the sheer chaos of it all. Whenever they reached a town there were all nationalities – French aviators, pitiful Austrians, German prisoners – penned into an orchard begging for bread and cigarettes, selling their helmets and belts:

One lad who spoke English well told us he had only left Berlin one month, he and his fellow prisoners were starving. They had all rather been shot than brought to Serbia to starve.

Then there was the indiscriminate nature of the suffering. Nurse Wren watched as a car went over the mountain, killing the Scottish nurses inside. A nun in a bullock wagon was accidentally shot in the lung by a Serbian soldier. When the Serbian soldiers travelling with Wren decided to steal a pony, the owner shot a soldier, the owner's son then shot a nun by accident and it all ended with the Serbs shooting the son.

As the weather worsened sleet turned to snow, which turned into blizzards. The Germans blocked their path so they had no alternative but to walk over the mountains. Nights were spent in stables, huddling together with soldiers of random nationalities for warmth, sleeping upright because there was no room. Everyone got dysentery. During the day they passed frozen bodies on the roadside and the snow was covered in blood from the bleeding feet of refugees, reduced to wearing sacking on their feet. They passed packhorses, too weak to carry on, which had been left to die.

They just stood looking meekly beside the path with no food. Snow covered everything too deeply for them to find any green food yet we could only push on, dreading a similar end.

The lack of food, and the hunt for it, was a constant theme. Sometimes they lived on maize bread with Nestlé's cream (Nurse Wren always carried her bread wrapped in a handkerchief in her coat to stop it from being stolen). Many days they walked tens of miles through the snow with no food at all. Even when they were given food, they were not able to cook it. A Turkish farmer gave them some precious meat, but it was three days before they could find somewhere to cook it. After leaving it overnight boiling in a pot, they woke up to find it had been stolen, with only the bare bones left. 'Still, at least we had slept well,' she wrote.

And that was what I took most from Nurse Wren – her resilience and resourcefulness. She never gave up, or slid into self-pity, or lost her faith in both humanity and God, and all done with a wry sense of humour.

Many times she praised the kindness of strangers and most of all, the Austrian Prisoners of War. One day, when the Ford car carrying the wounded got stuck in the snow and the chauffeur 'lost his mind', Nurse Wren walked three miles to the nearest village to borrow some oxen. Surly villagers refused her but after walking another mile she came across ten Austrian Prisoners of War, who offered to come and help. They got the car out, but all Wren's party could spare was a penny each, yet the Austrians were quite satisfied.

Indeed the kindness shown us by the Austrian prisoners all through our journey, allowing us to use

their camp fires, often holding our billycans on sticks
to boil them quickly for us, knowing we had nothing
to give them in return was most astonishing.

When her boots started to fall apart she commandeered
some slippers.

I managed to annex a pair of bedroom slippers which
I securely tied over my boots. They were pale blue.
Never did my bedroom slippers do such good service
before, soon they had frozen securely on.

When they eventually reached a town, Nurse Wren
and a few of her nursing companions were taken to the
house of a local Turkish official. She delighted in telling
of the glee of his many wives at meeting these foreign
women. The Turk talked to them through a brazier and
passed them food and cigarettes. The wives, meanwhile,
settled down to watch them undress and get into a clean
bed. Nurse Wren was mortified by the state of her pest-
encrusted clothes.

We had certainly been in some difficult positions, but
none quite so distressing as this, not having removed
our clothes for fifteen days.

When they finally got a first glimpse of the coast, it seemed
too good to be true. She sat down and gazed at the sea,

enjoying thoughts of home. Unfortunately the boat they were supposed to escape in was sunk in the harbour by German bombs. But hearing a rumour of another boat further up the coast, she decided to take the risk and walked another three days. The Italian captain was eventually persuaded to take her and she spent the night crossing the Adriatic standing upright in the forecastle, rolling with the waves and being rained on. On arrival at Brindisi she said she made a 'sorry spectacle'.

> *Up the street we ran, clutching our first white bread. Only those who have eaten maize bread for nearly nine weeks can realise the joy of a freshly baked loaf of white bread. The amazement of the people of Brindisi was amusing. Such a worthy company, in all kinds of attire, rushing through these delightfully clean and peaceful streets, must give them a very queer impression of the usual quiet people of Great Britain.*

She eventually reached Southampton on 23 December, just in time for Christmas.

At this point Nurse Wren quoted a prayer she found inside a book,

> *Father, who watchest in the silent heaven,*
> *knowing the sight, bidding me know it, yet*
> *Unconquerably silent, till I choose.*
> *Oh! In dizzying, weary to and fro,*

And counter-winds of question, in the blank
And shoreless void of doubt, where stares a soul,
Let me not err, Father of souls, not err
Thou wilt not speak, Yea, Lord, but let thy hand
Bar the false path in silence.

I closed the book and put it down. It seemed to be a prayer for me too. I had definitely been in the shoreless void of doubt and for the moment the Lord was silent; but was he barring the false path with Sister Alice's kind visit and the gift of Nurse Wren's diary?

The next day I took the diary back to Sister Alice.

'What did you think of it, my child?' she asked.

'I suppose I was amazed at Nurse Wren's resilience. The dreadful things she experienced and witnessed never seemed to shake her belief in God and humanity.'

'Or her vocation. What her diary doesn't tell you is that as soon as she got back she volunteered to go out to the front again and a few months later she was in Corfu.'

'Well, it certainly puts my doubts into perspective.'

'Indeed, child. Sometimes we have to accept our feelings are not relevant compared to what God is calling us to do.'

I nodded. The next day I went back to work. Whatever doubts Cecilia had had about her vocation, mine had vanished.

CHAPTER SEVEN

AN UNEXPECTED ARRIVAL AND AN EXPECTED DEPARTURE

By 1965 I was approaching the moment where I had to ask to be considered for life profession. If I'm honest, I was avoiding much serious thought about it. I was happy with the status quo, living in the Mission House and working as a midwife in Poplar, and with Cecilia's abrupt departure soon after taking her life vows in mind, I was anxious about rocking my own vocational boat. However, an unexpected arrival started to rock it anyway.

At half-past four one morning the doorbell of the Mission House clanged loudly and sent echoes round the House. As usual, one of the pupil midwives was on call. Today it was Brenda's turn. She opened the heavy Mission House door and looked out – there was no one there. She closed it again. A few minutes later the bell went again. By now I was awake and wondering what was going on; so I put on my dressing gown and slippers and made my way downstairs. Brenda was opening the door. This time she noticed a bundle on the steps and bent down to have a look.

'Good Lord!' she cried. 'It's a baby.'

I rushed down the stairs. Brenda picked up the bundle and there, wrapped up all snuggly, was a very new, pink, baby.

'Goodness!' I exclaimed. 'Someone has left it here. They must still be around. Check the baby, I'm going to find them.'

I left poor Brenda holding the baby and dashed out into the street. I looked left, right and across the square – there was absolutely no one to be seen. It was peaceful in the early morning light and all I could hear was birdsong. I hurried on, breathless and heart pounding, still in my dressing gown and slippers, and ran round the square. Then I did a crazy circuit of the streets around. I saw no one except for the odd docker or casual labourer, flat caps on, cigarettes in mouths, off to start the day looking for work. I was frustrated. Whoever had left the baby must be close by because they had been watching to make sure we found the baby, otherwise the bell wouldn't have rung a second time. However, as the streets of Poplar started to fill up with men on their way to work, I began to feel self-conscious about my lack of attire and had to admit defeat.

When I got back to the Mission House there was no one about. I went into the kitchen to find the entire household staring silently at a baby lying in the middle of the table. Once again I was reminded of the nativity scene; although this time, in the place of the manger, there was a table. Were we the shepherds or the wise men, or just the animals? Sister Dorothy interrupted my reverie.

'Look at us all. A bunch of midwives and none of us has a clue what to do.'

We giggled. This seemed to spur Sister Ruth into action.

'I suppose, Sister Catherine Mary, the fact that you have returned unaccompanied means that your search for the owner of this child has proved fruitless?'

I nodded.

'In which case I would like to welcome him to the world.'

'A boy?' I mouthed to Sister Alice standing next to me. She nodded.

With her expert midwife hands Sister Ruth picked him up and cradled him close. For once her inscrutable mask slipped and she looked serenely maternal. It was heart-warming to see Our Lady of Mystery transformed into the Virgin Mother.

'We do not know the name your mother would have given you, but as you have been handed into our care I would like to name you John Divine after our patron saint. As with every child, you have come from love and are welcomed with love, God's love. You may be separated for some time, maybe forever, from the mother who gave birth to you, but the Father who created you is always with you and His love will never fail. This greatest and eternal love will be given to you, John Divine, through us for as long as you stay with us. Sisters, shall we pray?'

As we bowed our heads, the medieval mystic, Julian of Norwich, came to my mind. One day as she held a hazelnut in the palm of her hand, she asked, 'What may this be?' and she received the answer, 'It is all that is made'. A hazelnut lasts forever because God loves it, 'And so have all things their beginning by the love of God'. Amen, I thought. And then I wondered whether Sister Ruth was about to grab some water from the sink and splash it over the baby John Divine's head. She didn't but I sort of wished she had. Instead she said this prayer, 'Dear Father, we can never know your plan. However we do trust in Your wisdom. We trust in Your wisdom for little John Divine here and we thank You for bringing him to us so that we can show him Your love. If it is Your will, we pray that John's mother can be found, but we accept it may not be the path You have chosen for him. Help us to love him and help him in any way we can. We pray that he thrives and is joyful, and that he feels that You are with him on his journey.

Dear Lord, you gave Jesus a family in Mary and Joseph and a home in Nazareth. We all need a home and a family so we pray that baby John is brought safely to a place that he can call home. Father Almighty, we give You our prayer. Amen.'

'Amen,' we all whispered back. I noticed Brenda was wiping a tear away from her eye.

Suddenly Sister Ruth's inscrutable face was back on and she was all business. 'Sister Alice, would you be so kind as to ring the police and then the social services and let them know of baby John's surprise arrival.'

'Brenda, I believe you have the day off today. I would be grateful if you could spend it tending to John. Of course you should find everything you need – nappies, bottles, blankets in the basement. Any problems myself and Sister Alice will be here. Sister Catherine Mary, could you find a box or a drawer we could use as a cradle for baby John?'

Sister Ruth handed the baby to Brenda and we all went off on our tasks. I emptied out my underwear drawer and took it downstairs to be Baby John's cradle. Brenda was tickled to be spending a day nursing a beautiful new baby. The police were called and a visit from social services booked, and the search for baby John Divine's family began.

The arrival of baby John Divine got me thinking. The Community of St John the Divine had been given many things over the years, but this was the first time we had ever been given a baby (and in fact the last). Why? It seemed curious. The Community of St John the Divine had first arrived in the East End in 1880 when the parish council of All Saints Church had written asking the Sisters to help nurse the poor of the parish. The Community immediately took over a small house in the square and were soon not only nursing the locals, but also delivering the babies of the 50,000 people who lived there.

Somewhat surprisingly the Sisters were not given a warm Cockney welcome. They were known locally as 'The Sisters of Misery'. Rocks were hurled at them by the local youth and there are even reports of rough women shouting rude words at them. I had an image of Sister Julia turning round and giving them an earful back, however there are no reports of any retaliation by the Sisters, so perhaps they were a slightly less feisty breed in those days. However, there was a rather dramatic turning point when the Sisters were sent for in the middle of the night to look after a 'rough Irish street woman'. She was nursed for five days and five nights until she died. Her friends sent a letter saying that the Sisters had looked after her 'as if she were your own sister'. To show their gratitude they clubbed together their pence and bought an illuminated card with 'God Bless this House' on the front. They presented it to the Sisters, saying it was all they could afford and 'only wished it was more'. After that the Sisters had no more trouble, indeed they quickly became a much-loved feature of the community.

By the time I reached the East End in the Sixties, the Sisters had been caring for the local families for four or more generations. The local policemen had to walk in groups of three at night for their own protection, but the Sisters could always travel alone. None of us had ever been assaulted or had anything stolen. I always felt the respect of the local people. Everywhere I went people would call out 'Hello, Sister'. If I ever needed the lavatory, I could knock on any door and I would be happily waved in. Perhaps, most importantly, in many cases we were delivering our fifth generation of local babies, so if a baby was going to be left anywhere, I would have thought the most obvious place would be on the steps of the Mission House.

So why was baby John Divine the first baby to be left on the doorstep? I was walking back from Evening Prayer pondering this very question when Sister Alice hurried up behind me (as much as was seemly for a Sister of a certain age to hurry) and, in a slightly conspiratorial fashion, whispered in my ear, 'Sister Catherine Mary, might I have a word?'

'Of course, Sister.'

'I have received a rather unusual invitation.'

'Oh yes?'

'It seems our good church warden,' she paused and I wondered whether she was being ironic – William Drake had only just been released from a short time inside for minor fraud, 'our good church warden has invited both of us to a party to celebrate his daughter Jacqueline's 21st birthday.'

'Oh.'

I didn't know quite what to say. Although we were loved by the community, we weren't usually invited to their parties.

'Yes, that was my initial reaction. But on reflection and prayer it seemed to make a certain sort of sense. You see, I delivered Jackie.'

Sister Alice then proceeded to tell me the story of how Jacqueline Drake had come into the world. Towards the end of the war a newly qualified Sister Alice was working as a midwife. She was summoned to deliver the second child of William and Bertha Drake. It was the middle of the afternoon and there was no sign of any Germans when she arrived, but then the labour started to drag on. Sister Alice was a bit surprised because Bertha's first delivery had been very straightforward. Then the sirens started. The family rushed off to the shelter, but what with all the excitement, Bertha was suddenly in the final stages of labour and couldn't be moved.

Bombs were dropping very close, bits of plaster were coming off the ceiling and they were in the dark. So there they were pushing, and panting, and suddenly there was a whistle and the most almighty explosion. The house next door was hit, the window blew in and Sister Alice was thrown on top of poor labouring Bertha. Just like a Charlie Chaplin movie, the huge window frame came crashing down around them, completely framing them on the bed. They were fine, plaster everywhere, but the baby came out two minutes later, screaming. It was a healthy girl.

Bertha called her Jackie because she popped out a bit like a jack-in-the-box. Sister Alice said a prayer and had a nip of the brandy she always carried for emergencies. And this *was* an emergency – she realised how shocked she was!

That same night one of the last V-2 bombs of the war hit the Community's Bow Lane house. The clergy and neighbours in the square rushed out and desperately dug through the rubble, but the only Sister left in there at the time, Sister Margery, was killed. Sister Alice then added, 'In a funny sort of a way I helped save Jackie's life, but she also saved mine. Because of course without her arrival keeping me out late, I would have been in the Bow Lane House too.'

Suddenly the invitation made perfect sense and it also explained why I had been invited. Six months before, I had delivered Jackie's first baby. Both Bertha and Jackie had fallen pregnant within a month of each other. This was not unusual for the time and the area. William and Bertha had married in their teens and so had their daughter Jackie. It seems rather strange now, but then it was quite common for nieces and nephews to be older than their aunts and uncles – a case of large families, early marriages and imperfect contraception. However, the modern world was creeping in. With Jackie still living at home (again not unusual in poor families) and two babies about to arrive, William had decided to invest in a telephone. They were still quite a novelty in Poplar houses. I used to arrive for my antenatal visits and find Bertha and Jackie sat in the front room staring at it. The phone had pride of place on a special little table right in the centre of the room. 'Oh dear, Phone, do ring,' Bertha would say longingly. Of course it never did because none of their family or friends had one.

Jackie's baby was due first and pretty much bang on the day I was summoned to go and deliver the first of the next generation of Drakes. It had been a straightforward pregnancy, but it was a difficult, hard labour. When Jackie's baby finally emerged he was blue and not breathing. In these situations I find my training automatically kicks in. The first step was to use a mucus extractor (like a tiny straw) to suck out any mucus from his nostrils. When this didn't spring him into life, I placed him on my lap and rubbed his back hard. This would usually elicite a gasp from the baby but new baby Drake was still lifeless and blue.

There was absolute silence in the room. Bertha was with us and I was aware she knew the seriousness of the situation. I tapped on his hand. For some reason this sometimes worked. But again, Baby Drake wasn't responding. Sometimes people held babies upside down by their feet or gently blew air through their lips. I wasn't convinced by either of these approaches. Instead I said, 'Bertha, can you reach in my bag and on the left you will find a small bottle.'

She waddled over, rummaged and quickly pulled out a small bottle of brandy. All of us midwives carried a bottle for just these kinds of emergencies. I opened it and placed a little bit of brandy under new baby Drake's tongue. Immediately he screwed up his eyes and started to squirm, and a couple of seconds later an angry yell filled the room.

'Thank the bloomin' Lord!' Bertha said.

'Is 'e goin' to be all right, Mum?' Jackie said, peering anxiously as I massaged baby Drake's back.

'Yes, sunshine, 'e is. Look at the beautiful little fella!'

Jackie promptly burst into tears and the tension in the room was broken.

'So,' said Sister Alice. 'What do you think about going to the party?'

'Well, I would rather like to go,' I said.

'Yes, indeed. I would rather like to go too.'

'But Sister Ruth?'

'Don't worry, I think it's best if I talk to her.'

The next day Sister Alice caught me in the corridor.

'Sister Catherine Mary, we have been given permission to go to the Drakes' party.'

'Oh really? How did you manage ...?'

'Ours is not to wonder why. There is only one thing you need to know – we have to be back in time for Compline.'

'Yes, yes, indeed, Sister.'

I bowed my head and bounced off to work, thrilled but feeling slightly nervous.

The party was taking place that weekend in the local British Legion club. Sister Alice and I first had to go to Evening Prayer so we were a little late for the party and among the last to arrive. The hall was full and a scene of happy smoke-filled chaos. Someone was making a racket on the piano and there was some rather raucous joining in. Lots of children were chasing around, getting into mischief and spoiling their best clothes, groups of young men stood in protective huddles, glasses of beer in hands, fags in mouths, talking to each other but eyeing the room, I presumed to spot female talent. The women were busy chasing the children, organising the food or gossiping. In places the generations mingled. There was a grandmother pulling what I presumed was her acutely embarrassed grandson onto the dance floor. At first no one really noticed us, but as people caught sight of the two Sisters in blue habits and white veils walk across the floor, there were lots of confused and amused double takes and nudges.

'All right, Mum. Love the fancy dress.'

To my horror one of the young men had grabbed Sister Alice's sleeve.

'Yeah. Sugar and spice kit. I love a bit of canoodling with a bit of chastity. Give us a hit and miss, your Reverence.'

At this point one of the young men planted a smacker right on Sister Alice's left cheek. A leery cheer went up from the group and everyone turned around. Sister Alice, pink to the very roots of her veil, took her arm firmly away from the young man's grasp and drew herself up.

'Sister Alice of the Community of St John the Divine. Very pleased to make your acquaintance.'

I was bracing myself for the young man's reply, but we were saved by William Drake pushing his way over to us.

'Oi, Charlie! Hands off the Sister, you great idiot!'

'Whoooo, Bill! If I'd known we was dressin' up, I'd 'av come as the Pope.'

'Leave it out! I told yer, this is Sister Alice. She's a nun, you idiot! She delivered our Jackie and this is Sister Catherine Mary and she did our Jackie's baby, and I'd appreciate it if yer gave 'em some respect.'

The young man, Charlie, looked at William and then at us and then back at William again, and then he took a deep breath and exhaled whistling through his teeth.

'Well, Sisters, my apologies. I'm just not used to seeing religion at a Moriarty.'

Sister Alice graciously bowed her head and said, 'Indeed. Well, Charlie, your apology is accepted, although I think it would be wise to ask permission before you kiss a lady next time.'

'Right yer are, Sister, right yer are. So I'm not goin' to Gypsy Nell then?'

'No, Charlie. You're not going to hell, not this time anyway …'

Everyone laughed and from then on the party went swimmingly. Charlie's terrible indiscretion had broken the ice and everyone wanted to talk to us, especially the women. They loved the opportunity to get a blow-by-blow account from the horse's mouth of the dramatic arrival of both Jackie and her baby son.

As I was introduced to the different guests I was struck by how inter-related they were. I was in the midst of a huge extended family, some of them related in different ways several times over. At one point Flossy grabbed my arm. She was a regular at church and I knew her well, in fact everyone knew Flossy well. She was William Drake's sister-in-law, but she was also Bertha's great-aunt, such was the complicated web of ties. Flossy was a force to be reckoned with. Only that year the Queen Mother had come to the rehallowing of St Botolph's Church in Aldgate. Outside wartime it was rare for royalty to come to the East End and everyone was talking about it. The service was to be a real event, with the Lord Mayor and the Bishop of London presiding, and attendance by special invitation only. For some reason Flossy had been expecting to be invited, but when an invitation failed to arrive, she got the hump and decided that she was going anyway. She turned up at St Boltoph's and managed to push her way past the stewards and curtsey just as the Queen Mother processed out, apparently saying, 'I do likes your 'ats, Your Majesty, but I don't thinks you should wear green.'

The first time I ever met her she was standing gazing at a new box, which had appeared at the back of the church. She pointed at it.

''ere, read this.'

It said, 'Donations for the discretion of the vicar'.

'What about his bleedin' indiscretions then?' she cackled.

The next week the vicar's mother came to the service. Flossy pulled my sleeve and gestured at her.

'She's all right but she ain't no oil painting, is she?' she said.

So Flossy was a bit of a handful, but I was impressed with however offensive she was (and she was), she was treated with love and respect. Her only children, her two sons, had been killed fighting in the war. Then during an air raid, Flossy went to the shelter but her husband stayed in the house. She got back to the house to find it had been bombed and her husband killed. But Flossy remained stoical and cheerful, and as I got to know her I noticed how her friends and family looked after her. Someone would always be sent to bring her to church and someone would always take her home. Whenever I called round, there was a visitor who had brought a piece of cake. She was a feature at any happening that involved a member of her large extended family. And Flossy wasn't unusual. The backbone of the area were the large extended families who had been there for generations and looked after each other.

Flossy looked me in the eye and asked somewhat slyly, 'So, Sister, I hears the stork brought you a special package this week.'

'Yes, indeed, Flossy.'

'I hears it's a little boy.'

'Yes, it is.'

'And he's healthy?'

'Yes.'

I was beginning to wonder why she was so interested. Then again Flossy was interested in everything going on.

'And has you found Mum yet?'

'No. The police are looking but absolutely no leads as yet.'

I paused and looked her in the eye.

'Flossy, do you know anything about the little boy?'

'I can't say as I do.'

'Come on, you know everything that goes on around here! This is your patch and don't pretend it isn't.'

'Well, yes, Sister, you can bleedin' well say that again.'

'So if there was anyone about to have a baby, or had had a baby or maybe even was a baby missing, you'd know about it, wouldn't you?'

'Well, Sister, puts it this way, I know everything that goes on with us.' She gestured around the hall. 'But I don't know everything what goes on with them, if you know what I mean.'

'Um ... not really.'

'Well, it's not just us, is it? There is peoples what pass through, if you gets me drift. Boats come, people gets off, they go about their business and then people gets back on again, and the boats go. Do ya' get what I mean?'

'Yes, I think I understand. So you think baby John must have been left by someone passing through?'

'Well, puts it this way, we looks after our own.'

She nodded towards one of Bertha's nieces, young Molly, although that wasn't her real name. Just the year before, Brenda, the pupil midwife, had been called out to a room for what she thought was going to be a first antenatal visit. What she found was 18-year-old Molly in the final stages of labour. Brenda had only been with us a month and had never delivered a baby on the district before. Moreover, Molly was lying in a bare room on a mattress with nothing else, not even a sheet on it. Brenda ran out into the street, looking desperately for a public telephone, so she called the Sisters for help. What she found instead was Mrs Hardy.

'Get back in there, luv. I'll sort it.'

Within minutes Mrs Hardy had managed to swing the Poplar matriarchy into action. Someone called the Mission House, someone else had managed to drag out of retirement what used to be known as the 'lying-in lady', who, in the days before midwives, would be called upon to deliver the local babies, and the others came flocking, bringing supplies of blankets and baby clothes and tea in a flask.

Back in the room, Brenda was putting on a brave face but clearly didn't have a clue what to do. The lying-in lady pushed past and took over. Soon a new baby was emerging into the world. There were gasps and claps all round. But Brenda, having recovered from the shock and relief of the birth, realised there were some serious questions to be asked. She took Mrs Hardy aside.

'Why was no one told about this baby? She's had no antenatal visits, no preparations have been made. I mean, there's not even any furniture here.'

'Hmmm. Well, it's placin' House to Lets on the bloody 'orses.'

'I'm sorry?'

'You's new round her, aren't ya', treacle? Gamblin'.'

'Gambling?'

'Yeah. That's 'er problem. She's been foolin' around trying to pay her debts and now she's got a lifetime one round her Gregory Peck. Daffy Girl! I'm gonna fetch her Mum. She's gonna 'ave something to say.'

Gambling was absolutely rife in the East End at the time. Everyone was at it and they bet on everything. Of course horses and cards were popular but the big thing was the dogs. To pay for it they would beg, borrow and steal. Whole houses' worth of furniture would end up at the pawnbrokers. Tragically, it was not unknown for young girls to try and pay back debts by sleeping with someone. It was never clear that this is what had happened to young Molly but that was certainly the rumour that went around. However, the reason Flossy had pointed at Molly was because the story had a relatively happy ending. While Molly received a good shouting at by her parents, her baby was immediately welcomed and absorbed into the family. Molly's Mum did most of the looking after but Molly's big sisters and aunts and Gran also joined in, and he became just another of the next generation. Molly went on to get a job and get married and start a new family. So Flossy was right – East Enders did look after their own.

Hurrying back with Sister Alice after the party, one part of my mind was anxious about being late for Compline, but the other part was thinking about baby John Divine. I came to the conclusion that the fact that he was the only baby that had ever been left with us was a reflection on the nature of the Community. I decided I felt a bit like a guest spider (small, not furry) in a large interlocking web. It was a web which covered the whole area and had lots and lots of threads, which were not neatly arranged in circles but messy – lots of threads connected to lots of other threads in illogical ways. Some threads were long, some short, but they were all connected lots of times. This meant that although the web looked fragile, it was actually very strong. If you landed in it, you would be held. If one thread broke there was always another one to pick you up. It meant that unexpected babies would not fall through the net. They would be caught and held in the web, the burden of their care usually being spread.

Thoughts about East End families put me in mind of my own family. They were only 30 minutes' bus ride away and yet I hadn't been to see them. Of course I wrote at least once a week and telephoned on birthdays and occasions, but I'd been in Poplar for over a year and I hadn't been home. I was avoiding it, but I wasn't sure why, although I thought it might have had something to do with that looming decision about taking my life vows.

Once I had become a novice I had to spend some years testing my vocation. We were supposed to live the life and see whether it was right for us, and truly find out whether God was calling us. These years of testing are seen as an opportunity to explore what each of the vows of poverty, chastity (or more rightly, consecrated celibacy) and obedience might mean for you personally and whether they felt right for you. People think that they mean no money, no sex and do as you're told. But in the years I had been with the Community I had come to see that consecrated celibacy is the most central vow. It is a consecrated celibacy where you give yourself to God in His service. It's about learning to love and it affects every level of your being. I had come to see that for me poverty was about stewardship and simplicity. It was about sharing God's gifts evenly and fairly, and living a simple life, of having only what is necessary in order to serve God. For me it was the easiest vow – a blessing, really – giving me freedom to concentrate on the things that are most important. Obedience was of course more difficult but I began to see it as being about listening to God and listening to those around me in order to find the common mind. The more time I spent living the religious life, the more it felt right and I was deeply grateful that I was able to express this in the world through my work as a midwife. I had a growing sense that I was in the right place, but I still didn't want to face taking the next irrevocable step.

However the week after the Drakes' party, the matter was taken out of my hands on a quick trip to the Mother House and a meeting with Mother Sarah Grace. Completely out of the blue she threw one simple question at me.

'Sister Catherine Mary, do you feel ready?'

The shock. I jolly well knew what she meant but I still asked.

'Ready for what, Mother?'

'You know what. So are you?'

I physically felt all a-quiver, but I managed to stammer out, 'Yes, Mother, I believe I am.'

'In which case, child, take your time but the next step is to write your application.'

I walked out, confused as to why, when faced with the question whether I was ready, I'd said 'Yes' when clearly 'No' would have been closer to where I was.

So I was sent away and expected to work on my application. Over the next few months, when I retired to my room 'Endurance', I sat at my little desk and looked at the empty page. I had to write a couple of sides of A4 charting my journey through faith and the reasons why I felt it was right for me now to take the next step. I prayed hard but nothing really came. I wondered whether going to see my family might clear my writer's block so I asked for a week's leave, which Sister Ruth happily granted, and climbed on the bus to Camden Town.

Coming back to Camden Town, I was struck by how it was rather mixed. Poplar was all just poverty, but Camden Town had pockets of prosperity and swagger. Some bits had grown rather fashionable – the large, beautiful Georgian houses had been done up while other bits had become more rundown and tatty. My road was looking tattier.

When I walked in the smell and colours of my home assaulted me in an unsettling way. In a way nothing had changed and then in another way everything had changed. There was the familiar smell of Mum's oil paints (she always had a picture on the go). Her other hobby – dressmaking – was also still very much in evidence. Dressmaking tools were scattered about, the tailor's dummy was in the corner of the kitchen with cloth draped over it; it made me smile. Mother gave me a peck on the cheek. It felt good to see her, but I felt a bit awkward; I didn't know where to put myself, or quite what to do. I didn't have a role or a routine. I had a cup of tea and a chat (again difficult, where to start? How to talk about a life that was so alien and based on a belief she didn't share?). In the end I excused myself, and went up to my old bedroom and put the battered old communal suitcase that all the Sisters shared on the bed. The bedroom seemed overcrowded. There wasn't that much furniture, but compared to the convent it seemed fussy, overblown, a bit extravagant. The flowery wallpaper gaudy, the trinkets wasteful. Coming back home put my present life in sharp relief.

Everyone was pleased to see me, but behind their smiles I could see a wariness, a slight hanging back when they hugged me. It revealed itself as I walked into the sitting room. My sister snapped, 'Walk properly, don't just glide.' The noise of the house assaulted me. There were people coming in and out, shouting and laughing.

Did they have to talk so loudly? It seemed unnecessary and selfish, and yet it wasn't. I had just got used to a contemplative life, where sound was seen as something to be used only where necessary. The radio was always on and the sound of the television filled the house in the evening and interfered with my prayers. I couldn't get used to the late nights as the family stayed up watching television or the late mornings. I used to be an owl but as a Sister you had to be a lark, up with the dawn chorus. My internal clock had readjusted. As a result after the first couple of nights at home, I felt tired with frazzled nerves and longed for a break and some order.

The next day I went down to breakfast and my little brother Harry (I say little, but by now he must have been 24) was sitting at the kitchen table with a friend. The friend looked aghast when I entered. Of course I was wearing my habit. Harry immediately clocked the look on his friend's face and said, 'Oh, meet my sister. You can kiss her, just don't get into the habit.'

They both burst out laughing. I could feel myself blushing. I knew that behind the joke Harry was embarrassed by me and I really didn't want to sit down and eat with them. I managed a quick cup of tea and piece of toast, and then I made my excuses and exited stage left, upstairs to the bedroom. I sat on the bed, tears of shame pricked my eyes, and then I felt guilty for being ashamed: I was only doing what I believed in. Why was that so embarrassing?

I closed my eyes and prayed. A picture of the disciple Peter came to mind and the cock crowing three times. The path to God was never easy for anyone. It wasn't supposed to be – we had to be tested. I thought of the early Christian martyrs and the fear, persecution and ostracising they had experienced. Was I so weak that a thoughtless joke could rattle me? I went to my wardrobe and from right at the back took out my old clothes – the best dress and two-piece suit I had saved in case I wanted to escape. I took off my habit and struggled into the dress. With its full skirt and tight bodice, it was hopelessly out of date. Everything in the streets was short and loose. It was also too tight and I could only get the zip done halfway up my back. I looked in the mirror: I looked ridiculous. I couldn't go back now. I was out of date, the world had moved on and the clothes didn't fit. The girl who had worn that dress to harmlessly flirt and drink a few glasses of something slightly alcoholic no longer existed. I had grown up and beyond. Then Mother walked in and I was mortified.

'Oh, Katie, what on earth are you doing?'

'Mother. Um … I'm just trying my old dress on. I don't know, really.'

'You funny thing! That's your party dress, isn't it? You used to look beautiful in it.'

'Mmmm. I look kind of ridiculous now.'

'Mmmmm. Yes.'

We both laughed and then I burst into tears.

'Oh, Katie. Come here.'

She sat on the bed and patted the space beside her. I sat down and she put her arm round me.

'Don't be upset by Harry. He doesn't mean it. He just doesn't know how to handle it. It's quite unusual to have a sister who's a nun.'

'I know.'

'We all love you and we are all proud of you.'

'Really?'

'Yes. I think we find it difficult to show. We're still getting used to it.'

'It's been more than seven years.'

'Yes, but we never see you. It's like you've died. We all miss you terribly.'

'But in a way I *have* died. And I've been reborn.'

She drew back from me and took her arm away from my waist.

'Katie Crisp, don't start talking to me about resurrection.'

'But I'm not Katie Crisp, I'm Sister Catherine Mary.'

Mother started to cry. She never cried, not even when Father died.

'There's no going back. I can't go back,' I said.

'I know. It's just I miss you.'

'You have to let me go. I've started on a journey I couldn't help and there's no going back.'

And before I knew it, I was saying it.

'I'm going to take my life vows.'

'I know. I had hoped you might come back but I can see now that you've already gone. Katie, I love you, we all do, and if it's what you want, we will support you.'

'It is, Mother, it is.'

We finished the conversation with a hug and the rest of the week was much easier.

When I got back to the Mission House I was told I needed to go straight out to visit old Flossy. While I had been away she'd had a heart attack and had been sent home from hospital because there was nothing more they could do for her. I was told she was comfortable but her end was very near, and I needed to go and sit with her. I wasn't surprised: she frequently had blackouts. In fact, only the Christmas before she had come to have dinner with us and just as we were about to go in and eat she fell down as if dead. As we peered anxiously over her face she opened an eye and said, 'Oh, you spoilt it!'

I arrived to find Flossy had already zipped herself up in a shroud, which she had purchased a couple of years before. It was a bit of a shock – I wondered whether I had arrived too late, but she opened one eye and said with a grin, 'Saves you havin' to do it, Sister,' and closed her eye again.

I sat with her as the day darkened and the room became lit by a solitary light. Her breathing grew shallower and eventually the breaths came further and further apart. I stroked her pale, fragile hand and prayed. I was struck with the similarities between helping someone to leave the world and helping someone enter it. Birth and death, two huge transition points in the soul's journey. It felt so important to be there alongside Flossy; to help her make this transition with courage and hope. I do believe that just as you can have a good birth, you can have a good death. It's important if you are with someone at these most profound moments of existence to be intuitive, to form a bond quickly, even if you have never met before so that you can say what needs to be said. (And of course hearing is the last sense to go, so even if it seems like they have sunk very low, it's important to keep on talking. Many is the time I have carried on talking when it seems they have gone to sleep and a slight squeeze to my hand will show they are still with us.)

It's important to assess where the person is on their spiritual journey, whether they have travelled to the destination they are supposed to reach and are therefore ready to die. And it's not necessarily got anything to do with how old they are. I've been present at the deaths of quite a few young people, who are ready to go and at peace, and similarly, older people who have lived many decades and yet are terrified. But old Flossy was ready to go; I sensed her peace and readiness to take the next step. I carried on praying and talking quietly to Flossy, telling her I loved her and how many people loved her, thanking her for being with us, telling her to have the courage for the next stage and my hope that she would soon see her sons and her husband again. I assured her she was loved and that her journey was going on. 'Can you see the light, Flossy? Walk towards the light.' This was the first of many times that I felt as if I was walking with the dying patient. I was walking alongside Flossy and I had to go as far as I could with her. But there came a point where I could go no further, but I had gone far enough that there were those on the horizon (angels, loved ones who have already died, I don't know), that she could see and they could see her and would be waiting for her, arms outstretched.

I have no idea if this is actually what happens, but this is what I like to think. Now, years later, I have met quite a few people who have had near-death experiences and all of them say they no longer fear death, that they go towards the light, feel an incredible peace and joy, and an awareness of the presence of others.

We can never start thinking about death soon enough. None of us knows when it will come, but we hurtle through life with our hands over our ears singing loudly. I've seen good deaths and I've seen bad deaths, and the good deaths are where a person has thought and prepared. Where they are surrounded by people who love them, they have found meaning in their lives, and made peace with their Maker; they have some sense of where they might be going. They have given instructions how they want to die and, most importantly, said the things they want to say to the people who matter to them.

I realised Flossy hadn't breathed for a while. Suddenly I felt alone, as if while I had been praying her soul had picked up its suitcase and quietly left the room for its next destination. I felt tremendously privileged to have sat beside her on this most important of journeys, zipped up in her shroud, totally ready for what was going to happen next. In that peaceful, darkening afternoon I was blessed with a sense of the human journey, from the dramatic moment we enter this world to the moment we exit it, and how important these moments are.

And when I got back to the Mission House I started to write my application to take my life vows.

About six months later we received word that baby John Divine had been adopted. After the conversation with Flossy, I hadn't been surprised that the search for his relations had proved fruitless. We continued to pray for John Divine for a long time after. Indeed, on the anniversary of the day he arrived on our doorstep, we often still say a prayer for him. He must be well into his forties by now and I guess no longer called John Divine, but I hope and pray he is living a good life and feeling the love of God.

He is a person we have never forgotten over the years.

CHAPTER EIGHT

THE WINDS OF CHANGE

I was amazed to discover during my nurses' training that every cell in a person's body is renewed within seven years. This means that there is not one bit of my body that now exists that was on this earth seven years ago. We are, literally, physically reborn many times during our lifetime. It's no wonder then that societies as a whole are never static. But sometimes the pace of change becomes more intense. Just as at critical points in a person's life – childhood, adolescence, pregnancy, old age – this rate of change speeds up, so the Sixties was one of those moments in this country's history when the pace of change became turbo-charged.

I became aware of this while doing my rounds on the district. The new tower blocks that were going up on the old bombsites or replacing the tenements instantly changed the whole nature of our area. Suddenly the material well-being of the Poplar housewife was transformed. There was an end to the communal outdoor privies, instead there was a lavatory and indeed a proper bathroom for every family. Out with rugs and lino, in came fitted carpets (they seemed the height of luxury!). The women of Poplar started to have things that their grandmothers and their mothers could only have dreamed of – washing machines, telephones, vacuum cleaners. But in the midst of this something was lost, something that money couldn't buy, something that might have been more precious.

I had an inkling of this the first time I visited Ivy Bucket in her flat in the new high-rise tower block by the Blackwall Tunnel. Before this Ivy had been living in what to an outside observer these days might look like something close to medieval squalor. The house was always a tip – dirt, dust, insects, you name it. There were clothes drying everywhere, plates piled up, broken toys on the floor, her countless cats and children getting under everyone's feet.

Because Ivy's friends and family lived in the surrounding streets (sister one door along, Mum the street behind, cousins on the corner) there was always another Cockney companion putting forward an opinion on every antenatal visit, and there had been quite a few because Ivy was on her fourth child. It felt overcrowded, but friendly. However, at the back of the house she always kept a special room for her newest baby. It was clean and warm, with a cot and perfectly pressed clothes all laid out neatly. I found it touching. As her fourth pregnancy advanced she received word that the council had found her a place in the brand new Balfour House tower block. Ivy was very excited.

'Bloody marvellous, Sister! Imagine, getting away from all this,' she said, sweeping her arm across her tiny, tatty kitchen, 'Everything brand new and even me very own loo.'

So for my next antenatal visit I had to cycle across the length of the district, which was no mean feat. The area we covered was a long ribbon stretching for miles. Gosh, it kept me fit, going backwards and forwards every day with my sturdy black bike and a bag complete with oxygen tank strapped to the side. Ivy's new flat was at the far end. When I got there I realised I hadn't a clue how to find it. The collection of high-rise tower blocks formed a rabbit warren of grey, dark concrete staircases. The streets were usually full of people; but this was a ghost town. Where was everybody?

I finally found Ivy's staircase but I was faced with a problem. How on earth was I going to get my equipment ten storeys up? And I didn't like leaving my bike. Normally I wouldn't think twice because our bikes never got stolen, but I sensed an unusual threat in the air and I didn't even carry a bicycle lock with me so I just had to prop it against a wall. I also felt self-conscious in my Sister's habit. It seemed to fit with the terraced houses but it looked ridiculous here. I picked up my equipment and looked around for a lift.

After a bit of wandering, I found the lift, but it wasn't working. I struggled back to the staircase and started the long climb up. I arrived rather ruffled and panting at Ivy Bucket's door. It wasn't very welcoming. No bell, no knocker, no window, just a number on a grey door. I rapped on it and Ivy opened the door, 'Come in, Sister. Oh lordy, what a heavy dirty slag! I bet you 'ad trouble getting that up the apples 'n pears.'

'Yes indeed, what happened to the lift?'

'Bleedin' thing is broken. It's been broken ever since we moved in. It ain't 'arf difficult getting up and down while I've been carryin' this.' Ivy pointed at her not-too-small bump.

'Yes, not designed for a pregnant lady. Designed by a man, of course – must be.'

'Too right, Sister. And 'ow on earth am I goin' to get the Fireman Sam and the chuffin' shopping up and down?'

'Oh gosh! Of course, the pram. That's a real problem. Why didn't they think of these things? Have you asked the council about the lifts?'

'Well, they won't fix 'em becos the kids play in them and breaks them again.'

'What?'

'I ask ya, what a rathead situation.'

I could see Ivy was getting worked up and I didn't blame her, but I was worried about her blood pressure.

'Well, the flat looks nice, Ivy.'

She smiled.

'Yes, Sister, it is. 'Ave a butcher's at this.'

She waddled through the small hall and flung open a door and switched on a light.

'Me very own bathroom, like the Queen.'

There was a small sink, bath and loo, all in white with new fluffy pedestal mats embracing the bottom of the ceramics. It didn't look like it had been used.

'And look at this, Sister.' She waddled through to the kitchen. A cooker; again so shiny and new and clean. Was she using it, I wondered?

After I had done my routine examination, Ivy seemed reluctant to let me go. She made me a cup of tea (with Carnation milk) and pressed a biscuit into my hand and nattered on. She seemed a bit lonely so I said, 'It seems very quiet, Ivy. Where are all your children? Shouldn't they be home from school by now?'

'Well yes, Sister. Thing is, they don't come straight home now. They miss their friends and there's nowhere for them to play. They're back down the street, I guess.'

'Oh. It does seem very quiet out there.'

'It's bleedin' quiet in 'ere and all.'

I suddenly realised her toddler was missing too.

'Where's Lizzie?'

'Oh, Mum's got her. She won't come 'ere 'cos she says she can't find me and she can't climb the stairs so I leaves her there.'

'Oh gosh, Ivy! This must be a bit difficult for you.'

'It is. I'm almost wishing I never came. I'm bleedin' lonely. Stan don't come home 'till late because he stays in the pub drinkin' with his china plates. He don't know no one round here.'

I nodded. The East End communities were so insular in those days that a trip to Whitechapel was seen as a bit of an event. Some people never left Poplar. It was what made the web so strong. But these new tower blocks were breaking up the threads of the web very quickly. Families were being split up and juggled around; new people moved in. The tower blocks were not conducive to people getting to know each other; and actually, people didn't want new friends, they wanted their old ones. It struck me that it took generations to build that sort of a community; it could only happen organically over time. But goodness, how quickly it could be dismantled. A community needed to live close to each other, constantly bumping into each other. Now geographical space was creating emotional distance. It was terribly sad.

Family ties were also loosening because women didn't need each other in the same way. Children, or rather the abundance of them, had kept women at home and relying on each other to help out. Of course there have always been ways of not having babies, coitus interruptus is the oldest form of contraception and condoms made out of animal intestines were being used by the early Egyptians. But these were either pretty ineffective or relied on the compliance of men, who let's face it, as they didn't have to look after the consequences, didn't have the same incentive to sort it out.

All this changed in 1961 when the contraceptive pill became available on prescription. At first it was given only to married women. They had to bring a letter from their vicar or some other such worthy to say that they were a suitable candidate to receive it, meaning they were respectable, married and in need of legitimately limiting their family numbers. But like an unstoppable force, once the water started to leak, the dam broke and soon thousands of women, married and unmarried, started to get the Pill. Within ten years a million women were using it. Now, for the first time, women had a highly effective form of contraception that didn't involve the cooperation of men and this meant that the birth rate dropped dramatically in places like Poplar.

Women were much more able to go out to work, and they did so because the traditional men's jobs in the docks were disappearing, and they needed the money. It also meant that without the threat of pregnancy women were able to have sex without getting married, so they started to marry later. Young Molly didn't have another baby for a long time after the one poor Brenda delivered. She carried on working and only started a family ten years later, when she finally married. This meant that the women didn't need each other's help in the same way. They didn't meet handing over small people; they were off in their places of work most of the time.

I noticed it on the streets. Fewer bumps, fewer prams, and less work for us. In the space of a few years the number of babies we delivered declined dramatically. Instead we had to learn new skills. Gradually, during the course of the Sixties, we started to routinely give advice about contraception as part of our post-natal care. At first it was something that I would bring up in conversation according to whether I felt it was an issue – for example, with a mother who already had five children. Faced with a mother who'd had two babies within 12 months of each other, I would say things like, 'You know you *can* get pregnant while you are breastfeeding, don't you?' (It's amazing how that myth persisted, and believe me, it *is* a myth!) Or if a woman had suffered damage I would caution her about resuming sexual relations before she had healed and then encourage her to insist that her husband was gentle (in those days so many women had to be given permission to be assertive with their husbands when it came to physical relations). But at some point in the mid Sixties it became one of the routine questions on our post-natal checklist, 'Have you thought about how you are going to prevent another pregnancy before you are ready?'

However, it became apparent that there was a growing need for family planning services, not only for those women who had just had babies, and that this was something it would be appropriate for us to provide. People often assume that because we are Sisters, we do not approve of contraception, but of course this is quite wrong. They are confusing us with nuns from the Roman Catholic Church, who will be guided to follow the papal line that artificial methods of contraception are against God's will. However, the Church of England has a different view of contraception, and having witnessed the suffering that came from backstreet abortions and the poverty that often came from having large families, we believed we could help.

In 1967 Sisters Alice and Dorothy were sent off on a training course and we started holding a family planning clinic one morning a week. It became a popular service, although one day a few years later, I was helping out when two young girls came in and looked rather shocked, stunned into silence in fact, to be facing a Sister in full habit in a family planning clinic. They sat there and stared at each other, blushing, and then stared at me. One of them nudged the other.

'You ask her.'

'No, *you* ask her.'

'No, *you* ask her.'

They sank back into a crippling embarrassed silence. I decided to put them out of their misery.

'Is there anything you'd like to ask me, girls?'

One of them piped up.

'Yes, miss. You see, we was wondering – is it true what they say, that you can use clingfilm as a contraceptive?'

'Well dear, that depends what you put it on, doesn't it?' I replied.

It felt rather a strange time to be doing something as medieval as becoming a nun when all around me the world was becoming frightfully post-modern. I was pondering the whole incongruity of it as I knelt in the chapel at the Mother House while I waited for news of my application to take my life vows. A full Chapter meeting of the Sisters had been called at my request, to deliberate my application. It didn't happen very often. I was the first applicant in years and it required every life-professed member of the Community to be present.

In a slightly party atmosphere we had all climbed on the train to Hastings. Well, I say party; I wasn't in a party mood. I just felt sick. In order to be accepted into a lifetime commitment, I had to be receive a majority of the vote and I couldn't for the life of me see the likes of Sister Julia giving me the nod. In fact I thought it might give her the utmost pleasure to trip me up just in front of the finishing line. Why were they taking so long? I looked at my watch. Actually it hadn't been that long, only half an hour. There was also a worrying precedent. The last Sister to apply had been turned down for first profession. Sister Victoria had been told she wasn't suitable and had had to leave pretty much straight away. We had since heard that she had very quickly met a vicar, married and was pregnant with her first child, which in a way seemed to bear out the wisdom of the Sisters' decision. But still, I had no desire to be out in the world looking for a husband and ending up as a vicar's wife. Walking on the moon seemed a more likely scenario. With this thought, I found my prayer.

'Dear Father, Please let the Sisters see what I see – that You are calling me to this religious life; that I want to serve You here and now in this way, that I want to give myself up fully to a life dedicated to You and to helping Your people on earth in the best way I know how.'

At this moment I felt a gentle hand on my shoulder. I jumped and swung round. It was Mother Sarah Grace.

'Oh, Mother, you startled me.'

Why, oh why, and how, oh how, did these Sisters manage to just appear, as if by magic?

'Sister Catherine Mary, we have finished discussing your application and have come to a decision. We'd like it if you could step into the Chapter.'

I looked at her face, desperately trying to read its expression. She seemed very serious, but then wasn't she always serious? I tried to recall when I had last seen our Reverend Mother smile, and I couldn't. I followed behind her through the corridors of the Mother House, wondering if the fact I had received no signal of affirmation from her, not a squeeze on the shoulder, or a helping hand to stand, meant something. It was a tortuous walk.

The Chapter meetings traditionally took place in a circular room underneath the chapel, which was reached by some winding narrow stone steps. The 22 Sisters were seated in a semicircle, with Mother Sarah Grace very much centre-stage, right in the middle. She gestured to me to stand in front of her and face the Sisters. There was silence. I felt like a gladiator standing in front of Caesar, waiting for the thumbs up or the thumbs down.

'Sister Catherine Mary, we have read your application and discussed it with the Community and we have voted.'

There was a pause. I felt myself swaying, my habit suddenly feeling enormously heavy.

'To accept your application and allow you to take your life vows. God bless you, Sister Catherine Mary. Welcome.'

The Emperor's thumb was up! There was a happy murmur around the circle and a little self-conscious round of applause. And then Sister Rachel got up and came over and embraced me, and she was quickly followed by Sister Alice, and then the whole team from Poplar. It was a joyful moment. I noticed Sister Julia hung back but that was no loss.

It was only a few years later when I was waiting to go into a Chapter meeting that I realised the quiet influence that the Mother Superior had. One of the more senior Sisters was quietly discussing a matter we were about to vote on and I heard her whisper to another Sister, 'Well, I don't agree but of course Mother wants this to go through', and there was nodding. The vote was carried and I was cross.

Surely the whole point of a vote was for the will of God to be carried through our collective conscience? Why have the vote otherwise? We may as well be living under a dictator. But then in the case of the election of a Sister perhaps it was a good thing because in the

Community even the most saintly of our number makes a few enemies. A religious community doesn't escape the human frailties of any other community on this earth.

A religious community also doesn't escape the winds of change that are blowing over everyone else. Yes, sometimes I wondered why I was taking a step back into the Dark Ages, but at other times it felt like there was a possibility I might find myself somewhere quite progressive. There were cracks rapidly appearing in the old order. The Christian Church was being shaken up by the Swinging Sixties, and I watched intently from the sidelines with real excitement.

It was customary for a significant period of time between the vote taking place and the actual ceremony to take life vows. I was given notice that I would have four months to prepare myself and reflect. At the same time as I was reflecting on my future, the Roman Catholic Church was engaged in a series of meetings reflecting on its own future, which would have a profound effect not only on the Roman Catholic Church itself, but also on the Anglican Church and therefore my life as well.

In 1958 John XXIII was elected Pope. A man with a vision and a mission, he saw the Roman Catholic Church as stuck in the past and imprisoned by tradition, with little room for a lively questioning faith that could grow and renew. Three months after his election, Pope John XXIII declared it was 'time to open the windows of the Church to let in some fresh air.' He called a Council to address the relationship of the Catholic Church with the modern world, to which one Cardinal said, 'This holy old boy doesn't realise what a hornet's nest he is stirring up.' This Council, known as Vatican II, began sitting in 1961 and was in its final stages in 1965 as I prepared to take my final vows. It called for the Catholic Church to return to its biblical roots and have a greater engagement with the modern world.

Part of its remit was to look at the lives of the religious orders. One decision which came out of the discussions was that there should be a greater recognition of the individual in religious life, meaning they should be able to fully participate in decisions affecting them. Along with this, religious orders had to take greater personal responsibility for ensuring God's justice in the world. It was radical and turned the existing order on its head – obliging religious communities to become more outward-looking and responsive to the world around them. I read the documents produced by the Council and I thought of Cecilia and how differently things might have turned out, had these principles been applied to her predicament.

I wasn't the only one excited about the news. There were reports of buses full of Catholic nuns going to special seminars and lectures to explore what this meant for their future. Results were immediate. The most obvious was the incredibly quick disappearance of the habit. Yes, some nuns remained in traditional habits (and still do), with full-length dresses and heavy veils, but within a few years the majority of Catholic nuns had adopted simple contemporary clothes. But the disappearance of the habit was just the visible sign of a much deeper change. In 1988, when the Cold War ended, and I watched the pictures of the Berlin Wall coming down on television, it reminded me of Vatican II. The Soviet Union broke up into lots of countries, with their own language, laws and ways of worshipping. Similarly, some of the larger Catholic orders started to break down and split into smaller, autonomous Communities.

With the breakdown of the Communist bloc came freedom of movement and expression. So the Catholic nuns were not only allowed, but urged, to mix with the world around them and go out to work. There was much greater freedom of expression and nuns were encouraged to continue their education. A whole host of them started university courses and a new breed of highly educated, theological, learned nuns was born. It really was revolutionary and as I watched, I was jumping up and down with excitement because I knew, I just *knew*, that what my Catholic sisters were getting today would be ours tomorrow.

However, my excitement was not shared by everyone in the Community. The split seemed to be between the older Sisters and the younger generation. The poor twins, Sister Clare and Sister Hope, were totally bewildered. Brought up by a loving, but domineering mother, they had no siblings and knew only each other and a mother who wanted to keep them safe from the dangerous, corrupting world outside. When they were still very young, she had encouraged them in the direction of the religious life.

Sisters Hope and Clare were wonderfully pure and naive. One year they took their annual holiday together and went on a coach trip around Italy. They made friends with an elderly spinster and after a long day's sightseeing decided to invite her into their hotel room for a cup of tea. They wrote a little note saying, 'Come to room 27, you know when, for you know what!'

Sister Clare put the note under the spinster's hotel-room door but when she didn't appear, Sister Clare realised she hadn't said whom the note was from. So she rushed back and put another note under the door, saying, 'By the way it's me, Sister Clare.'

But the lady still didn't appear. So Sister Hope asked, 'What room did you deliver the note to, dear?'

'Well, number 44, of course.'

'Oh well, that's why she's not here. She's in 54.'

Sister Clare dashed back to room 44 and banged on the door. It opened straight away and she found herself facing a distinguished elderly gentleman holding her notes. 'Are these yours?' he asked.

'Yes, they are, bless you,' she said and took them from him.

*

When she recounted the story to us later she revealed, 'The strange thing is he kept on winking at me after that. Funny man!'

The next year the Sisters decided to fulfill a lifetime's ambition to go and visit the Holy Land. As they went through the strict Customs on the return journey from Israel, Sister Hope was taken aside by an armed guard.

'Is this your suitcase?' he asked, pointing at the bag she was carrying.

'No,' she said, which of course strictly speaking, it wasn't. It was the communal suitcase we all took turns in using whenever we went on holiday. However, this set in motion an enormous security alert and delayed their aeroplane, and all the passengers waiting for it, by two hours.

For Sisters Clare and Hope, now in their sixties, the traditional way of life of a Sister was a comfort blanket; it meant security. I saw it, at its worst, as a way of keeping them as children; they never had to make a decision or take responsibility for themselves.

One day, busy with our needlework in the communal sitting room of the Mission House, we discussed the changes brought by Vatican II and Sister Clare piped up.

'Poor ladies, I shall pray for them – to have to give up their habits and move out of their houses. I couldn't bear it.' She shook her head.

'No, indeed. I shall be praying for them. God forbid anything like that should happen to us,' Sister Hope nodded in agreement.

I waded in.

'But I don't think that's what's going to happen. Isn't it about choice, so each Sister is more able to follow her own path as she feels called within the Community?'

'But how would we know which way to go? That is for the Mother Superior to decide,' said Sister Hope.

'And how does she decide – through prayer. Through listening to God. Isn't that what we are supposed to be doing all through the day?'

'But isn't that the whole point, child, it isn't clear?' Sister Ruth said, stepping in and looking at the twins.

Sister Julia, seething at the other end of the table, could hold back no longer.

'Muddle is the work of the devil. It is clear and it couldn't be clearer we have all taken a vow of obedience. All this talk of personal journeys, people's wants and desires taking precedence over the wishes of their Community; Sisters being consulted and asked their opinion over what they do next. Absolute rubbish! No, worse than rubbish – a slippery slope down. It's the will of the individual getting in the way of the will of God. Obedience is never negotiable, it is a state of grace.'

Now I was the one who was seething.

'And who exactly determines what is the will of God? What if, after constant prayer and contemplation, you feel God is taking you in a direction that your superiors don't agree with?'

'Then you ask God's forgiveness.'

'Do you think that's what Mother Caroline did when the Bishop of London told her to resign and she refused?'

There was a stunned silence in the room. I caught sight of Sister Alice trying to smother a smile. I'd got Sister Julia now and everyone knew it.

Mother Caroline is perhaps the most revered and beloved Mother Superior in the history of our Community. She was Mother Mary Jones' successor and led the Order for 20 years, through its biggest period of expansion and transformation. Though a quiet, gentle lady, she was highly religious, principled and determined. Her deputy, Sister Aimee, however, was a different matter altogether. She was appointed matron in charge of King's College Hospital and immediately came to blows with the hospital authorities over such small matters as beef tea and the washing of linen.

Sister Aimee was a strong disciplinarian and saw wickedness in even the most innocent exchanges between her charges and the male staff and patients. She introduced extreme rules: for example, no male medical officer was allowed to enter female wards during the hours of darkness. There followed a decade of trouble where the Sisters became quite unpopular and the hospital and the St John's Council asked for Sister Aimee to be removed. Mother Caroline refused, perhaps because she herself had been trained as a nurse under Sister's Aimee's care. It all came to a head in 1882, when Sister Aimee made a 'vile accusation' against one of the doctors, who she believed had manhandled one of her nurses. The accusation was proved to be false but Sister Aimee refused to retract or apologise. The hospital withdrew their contract with the St John's Community and the Council sacked Sister Aimee. But the Sisters and nurses under the leadership of Mother Caroline refused to leave the hospital. Instead they demanded the removal of the Council and to set up a Council of their own with Mother Caroline at the head and the Sisters in Chapter governing themselves.

The hospital chairman, Lord Francis Hervey, ordered the doors to the hospital to be locked against them, not knowing that the Sisters were already in there and he had effectively locked them in. There then ensued a three-day sit-in, with the nurses and Sisters refusing to leave. This is perhaps the first instance of a female sit-in in the Western world, a marvellous example of principled disobedience and a prototype for all the Sixties sit-ins that were about to take place. In the end the Sisters were persuaded to leave the hospital, but they also left the order and set up their own self-governing Community, with Mother Caroline in sole charge.

And so the new Community of St John the Divine was born. The old order struggled on with a skeleton staff, but was disbanded a few years later. The Sisters never again nursed at King's but from then on, their work was centred on the East End and Southeast London. But probably most importantly, they were free from their male Council and the authority that had always held them back from the more spiritual and devout lives they wanted to live.

Sister Julia could not argue against the heroic example of our beloved Mother Caroline, but she had to have the last word.

'What nonsense! It will have a sticky end, you mark my words. They'll be calling for women priests next!'

'And what if they did, Sister? What if they did?' I asked. 'What would be wrong with that?'

There was a gasp of horror from the twins in the corner. Sister Ruth decided this conversation had gone far enough.

'I think we can leave it there, Sister Catherine Mary. You have proved the point that our Community does indeed contain many different points of view. However, the important thing is that we come together in unity, that the things we agree on are greater than the things we disagree on, and we strive unceasingly to build on these, rather than widen the gap between us.'

For now, I accepted the calming words of Sister Ruth but I was determined not to be left out of any chance of progress. I thought it might indeed be possible to square the circle of religious life with the modern world and Vatican II had illuminated a path.

One of the developments to come out of the Vatican Council was a reaching out to other denominations and faiths. Suddenly, there were opportunities for us to go to meetings and seminars with our Roman Catholic counterparts. The week before I was due to make my vows, I had the opportunity to attend just such a meeting. The subject was how different Christian churches might work more closely together.

I was surrounded by Sisters who looked like my aunts – sensible shoes, pleated skirts, blouses and cardigans; short, neat, grey or white hair – the only clue to their profession being the large cross that hung from a long chain around each of their necks and the ring on their right hands. The feel of the gathering was very different to how it would have been, had it been full of Sisters in habits.

We broke in the afternoon for coffee and chat. As I stood in the corner of the room, I was a bit stuck. I am a natural mingler but usually a Sister's habit offered an easy opening line. For example, 'So, you come from the Community of St Clare, how is Mother Jane?' or 'I've been very interested in the work that the Sisters of St Margaret's are doing in Hackney', or 'I hear that the Sacred Heart are opening a new house in Manchester? Is Father Michael still the chaplain at your Mother House?' And off I would go. Now I looked around the room of sensibly-clad Sisters and found I had no bearings. I also felt rather self-conscious, being one of the only Sisters still in a habit. Suddenly, being a member of the Church of England felt rather regressive. Luckily, I was saved by the approach of a smiley Sister in navy blue cardigan and skirt, hair in a bun, glasses on her nose and a large wooden cross hanging from her neck.

'Hello, are you from the Community of St John the Divine?'

'Yes, I am. Sister Catherine Mary.' I held out my hand.

'Sister Sophia, Daughters of St Paul. I recognised the habit.'

'Yes, I'm in a bit of a minority here.'

'But such a wonderful habit, a beautiful blue!'

'Hyacinth, darling.'

'I'm sorry?'

I laughed.

'I used to work in the nursing home at our Mother House and one of the patients used to call out, "Hyacinth, darling".'

Now Sister Sophia laughed.

'You know, I always thought you had the best habit. If I was to wear any, I'd like to wear yours.'

'But you aren't wearing one. What's it like to be in mufti?'

'Well, at first I felt rather exposed and it was rather difficult to purchase a wardrobe. It used to take me a long time to choose what to wear in the morning but now I think it's rather wonderful.'

'Yes?'

'It means you have to work harder. You can't hide behind it. The barrier is down, people judge you more on yourself rather than your uniform. It takes more courage but in the end you make a better connection, a more authentic connection, be that with your Sisters, or with other members of the religious life like yourself, but especially in the wider community.'

I paused for a moment and thought.

'Yes, I can see that.'

'There have been so many changes. We are in freefall but it feels like a creative freefall.'

'That sounds rather exciting.'

'Well, I think there is a fundamental difference between Roman Catholic and Anglican Communities. Most of our Sisters have become nuns for reasons of their family background, tradition, because a lady of the family always did become a nun. In your case you have made a choice based on conviction alone.'

She gave a mischievous grin.

'Really?'

'Really. You only have to look at how many of our Sisters are leaving now to know that this was a path not of true vocation but of earthly considerations.'

It was true. In the years following Vatican II many nuns left their Communities, unable to cope with the change.

So there I was, preparing to join a way of life that most other people seemed to be fleeing from. The next day I started my obligatory four-day retreat before taking my vows. As I wandered through the woods surrounding the Mother House between my long hours of prayer, I pondered the seminar and it seemed to me that, as is often the case, the most profound bit of the day was not the formal agenda, but the encounter round the edges. For me, God was at work in my meeting with Sister Sophia. We were not diluted, I was called and I was called into a life that was changing and opening up. There were opportunities to bring God closer to the world and part of my calling was not to be a barrier to the winds of change but to go with the spirit and take down the barriers, add my own breath and life to it. God was moving and taking me with Him.

My life profession was to take place in the middle of the early morning Eucharist in the chapel at the Mother House in Hastings. I couldn't quite believe that because it started at 6.30 a.m. It would all be over by breakfast. 'The Bishop of Chichester is having an early start,' I thought to myself as I removed the silver Sister's ring from my right hand and put on my new habit. I was having a late start – I hadn't slept, but had spent all night in prayer.

In the chapel the service ran smoothly as it did every day, the familiarity of the words seeming too casual for the step I was about to take. But after the Gospel reading, it all started to happen. I was asked to step forward, the Bishop asked me a series of questions and I read my 'Declaration of Profession', which was signed and witnessed, and which I then placed on the altar. My signature was shaky; Mother Sarah Grace's much more firm. Then Mother Sarah Grace solemnly put a girdle around my waist that had three knots in it, symbolising the three vows of poverty, consecrated celibacy and obedience. The Bishop placed a gold ring on my right hand to be an outward symbol of my consecration to Christ and someone gave me a bunch of three white carnations symbolising my vows.

I stood there feeling awkward and thought, 'these will have to go', and then wondered why I was having the thought. Then unbidden the words 'revolution from within' came into my head and I felt guilty. It was as if no sooner did I make what was supposed to be the final step up the ladder then a whole new radical subversive one was opening up. When the service was over, I quietly went round to the side chapel and placed the carnations in the vase in front of the Statue of the Virgin Mary. There, as the early morning sun sent a shaft of light onto my head, I made my own little pact with the Divine: 'I'm going to work to take down all those barriers that come between me and You, I promise.'

A few years later I saw Ivy Bucket in the chemist's, but she wasn't in the queue: she was in a uniform, standing behind the till.

'Oh, hello, Ivy. What are you doing here?' I asked, intrigued.

'Morning, Sister, I've got a job.'

'Oh!'

'Yes. I was fed up sat in that bleedin' tower block all on my ownsome.'

'Good for you!'

'Yes, well, the kids are all at school and as you know, I'm not going to get up in the Pudding Club again.'

She gave me a wink.

'I've got me own bread and honey now and if I make it, I keeps it, and he can't blow it on the dogs.'

I took another look at Ivy. Her hair was tidy and had been cut in a fashionable bob – in fact, it might have even changed colour slightly – and she was wearing pale pink lipstick and eyeliner. She was looking years younger.

'You look very well, Ivy. Work is obviously suiting you.'

'Oh, it is, Sister! It's good to get out and meet new people. I've got a whole new lease of life.'

'Indeed, indeed! God bless progress, eh?'

'Yes, Sister, thank the Lord!'

The next thing I heard, she'd run off with the chemist …

CHAPTER NINE

AN UNEXPECTED JOURNEY

'You Can't Always Get What You Want,' is a famous Rolling Stones song. The lyrics then go on to point out that if you try, then you do sometimes get what you need. I heard the song playing on the radio in many of the houses I visited at this time in my life, and it never failed to put a wry smile on my face. Indeed, Amen.

In my first month at the Community I had been taken aside by Mother Sarah Grace and given a special mission.

'Sister Catherine Mary, this Community only survives and thrives through its members. We are a family and like all families, we need a new generation in order to grow and prosper, and prevent the Community from dying out. Of course we all regularly pray to the Lord to send new members to us. However, it is the special job of our newest addition to pray with great earnest for a new Sister. I want you to apply yourself with diligence to this task,' she said, before adding seriously, 'Do you understand, my child?'

I nodded obediently and applied myself by including in my prayers every day without fail the request for a new recruit. But as the days turned to years and no one turned up (or at least no one who stayed), veiled comments about the lack of interest from the outside world began to seem like a personal reproach; as if I wasn't praying hard enough or in the right way. It wasn't through lack of desire; I was only too aware that since Cecilia had left, the nearest Sister in age to me was 15 years older. I longed to sit at the table with someone who had at least been born within ten years of me. It was fun to have the pupil midwives around, but I could only join in and get close to them to a certain extent; my habit created a real boundary. Of course it would also be something of a relief not to be the lowest in the religious pecking order.

There were some false dawns. Word would get round that someone with an interest in the religious life was on her way. I used to get quite excited, but after a while I learned not to get my hopes up. People came and went. Some stayed a few months, others a couple of years, but for different reasons they all turned out not to be called to the religious life. A couple left of their own accord, one was ill, and then there were a couple who were gently told they were not suitable because it wasn't right for them.

The Community of St John the Divine had never been large. Even at its largest in the 1930s there had only ever been 30 or so Sisters. Our Community only wanted people they believed were called. There was one person who stayed for quite a while, but despite her intelligence and religious commitment, she found it difficult to move among us. There were arguments and atmospheres, and she was gently advised that life in Community was not for her. She regularly applied to rejoin, but her requests were always turned down. I began to lose hope, but eventually someone came to test their vocation who did stay.

Sister Ruth took me aside, looking almost excited.

'Next week we have a novice coming to Poplar! Yes, Marie-Louise will be joining us.'

She paused as if for dramatic effect.

'She has started her novitiate at the Mother House and Mother Sarah Grace has asked that she start her midwifery training with us. She will be spending a couple of weeks here before going to the London Lying-In Hospital for her Part One and of course will then return here to complete Part Two. I would like you to look after her for the next couple of weeks – show her around, take her on your rounds with you. Take care of her, she shows great promise.'

'Yes, of course, Sister.'

There was another pause and then she said something a little off piste.

'You must be so pleased. Well done!'

In that sentence Sister Ruth confirmed everything that I had suspected, that somehow in a cosmic sense I was being held responsible for the recruitment process. No one said anything directly, but over the coming few days as the Sisters prepared for the new arrival, I could sense that they were more excited than usual: they thought she was actually going to stay.

My first impression of Marie-Louise was positive. She was a pale, slender young woman, with rather piercing blue eyes. We went for a walk around the district, ostensibly to help her get a feel for the place; really, it was so we could get a feel for each other. She immediately started to ask me questions, the sort of questions she couldn't really put to our Reverend Mother, like 'So what's it like being in the Community?', 'Are they really strict?', 'What do you do every day?', 'Do you like being a midwife?', 'Do you ever get sick of praying?' (that last question made me sit up a bit!). I was impressed, though.

They were proper big questions, important – the sort of questions you should ask if you are seriously thinking of making this your life. But at the end of our walk I was also left with a feeling that I hadn't really managed to get a feel for her. There was something elusive. A bit like herding cats: when I was asking the big questions like 'Why the religious life?', 'Why the Community of St John's?', I realised she had managed to slip through my fingers without giving any real answers or indeed anything of herself away, despite the fact that I felt I had been open and honest with her.

I was left feeling a bit short-changed, especially as I was quite longing to connect and encounter someone new.

Later on I came to realise Marie-Louise's natural reserve was not coldness but shyness. But at that moment while yes, I did think she might well stay, I was left feeling the Cecilia gap was not about to be closed any time soon, or so I thought. Sometimes things happen when you are looking the other way.

The local clergy often visited us at the Mission House. They would pop in, sometimes stay for dinner, and we were often invited to their services or we had joint services. Our Bishop encouraged us to feel like we were all one big extended family. A particular vicar, let's call him Father Ian, was a frequent visitor to the Mission House. He was in charge of a particularly troublesome parish in our diocese, and he also struggled with his own personal demons. A difficult childhood of abandonment had left him anxious and prone to depression; he couldn't sleep at night.

Father Ian was quite attractive, with rather striking green eyes (the tiredness and pain behind them only added to their appeal), wavy chestnut hair and a large, athletic frame (not having the custody of the eyes, one does look at faces and therefore human thoughts about the nature of the other in front of us cannot help but occur!). But still I didn't think it was any accident that he hadn't married; as I said, he had personal problems. We had always got on well, though. For me, it was just such a joy to be around someone religious and relatively young (witness my excitement at the arrival of Marie-Louise). Then one day he asked to speak to me privately.

I took him into the Community Room, which happened to be empty; shut the door and motioned to the chair next to the unused piano. He sat down, leaned forward, and ran his fingers through his hair with an expression approaching anguish.

'Sister Catherine Mary, I find myself in a difficult position. I'm wrestling and struggling with some issues, and I don't know who to talk to.'

'Oh well, I'm sure the Bishop …'

'No, I've tried. While I have the utmost respect for the Bishop, I find it difficult to talk about matters that aren't strictly spiritual or connected to parish affairs.'

'Oh! Yes, well I can see how that might be a problem, but your spiritual director?'

'I think the Sisters do not have choice over their spiritual director, either.'

He gave me a wry, almost cheeky smile. A picture of the chaplain came to mind, so I said, 'Yes, indeed, Father Ian, I understand completely. How can I help?'

His face immediately crumpled and he put his head in his hands. He told me how his warring parishioners were threatening his already fragile self-confidence and turning his thoughts to very dark places. I felt a wave of concern and a desire to reach out to him. For a long time I had been practising having an openness to the other and a heart ready to give in love. Every day, as much as possible, I tried to extend the huge love I felt from my God to those around me, and I felt it all too easy to extend this love to this tortured, beautiful soul. So that afternoon was the beginning of a different relationship between Father Ian and me. He started to visit me regularly and I visited him in his parish and even cooked for him sometimes. Standing at his stove with an apron around my waist as he chatted to me sat at the kitchen table, it felt comfortable and natural, actually amazingly comfortable, like we had been doing this all our lives. He invited me to a couple of religious talks and services. I began to miss him when he didn't appear and find him creeping into my head when I was out and about, delivering babies. When I heard the doorbell ring, my heart leapt and I waited with butterflies in my stomach, listening in case there might be footsteps approaching to tell me that I had a visitor.

It was a kind of madness, like an infection. He'd got under my skin in a way no man had ever done. When I looked into those green eyes I felt a connection, like I could see his soul and he could see mine. For the first time I felt as if I was seen for myself; not Sister Catherine Mary, but Katie Crisp, a younger, more human person. I experienced a whole host of emotions and a depth of feeling I didn't know I possessed. It was powerful and seductive and terrifying. These emotions weren't just in my mind, but expressed themselves in my body too. My heart missed a beat when I saw him in the distance, I felt physical pain when he didn't appear, thoughts of him made my stomach lurch as if I was turning a loop on a rollercoaster. I missed him.

One day he took my hand and pressed my ring. I felt a shock run through my body. I knew I should gently remove my hand from his touch, but I didn't; instead, somewhat disingenuously, I pretended not to notice he was still holding onto it.

Were these feelings mutual? He never said anything but he kept looking for me and finding me. One day he quoted part of a line from a poem by W. B. Yeats at me, 'Tread softly on my dreams'. Would he have done this if he had known I knew the rest of the poem only too well? It is beautiful love poem, the sort that Mother Sarah Grace would have had removed from the library of the Mother House for being 'emotional'.

> But I, being poor, have only my dreams;
> I have spread my dreams under your feet;
> Tread softly because you tread on my dreams.

Another day he said to me, 'Catherine, no one understands me the way you do. I have never met anyone like you. You are so special, you light up my world. I thank God that He's brought you to me.'

But had He? Or was it someone darker, the other bloke, the fallen angel? Sometimes it felt pure heaven-sent and sometimes something much more earthy and tempting and wrong. And actually, the more I fell under the spell of Father Ian's seductive company, the more it felt wrong.

Every year we had a Service of Thanksgiving for the work of the Diocese. All the local clergy would gather and the Bishop would preside. Everyone would be in good spirits; it was a coming together, a happy day. But this year I was aware of a difference: I was distracted, looking over my shoulder; indeed looking for him. And that whole service I was aware that he was sitting just a few rows in front of me and instead of watching the Bishop, I was looking at the back of his neck. By the time we got to the blessing I hadn't managed to say anything meaningful to my God except, 'Why now God, why tempt me now, when I have just taken my final vows?'

Father Ian was creeping into my prayers and distracting me, and it was then that I knew he was coming between me and God, and I was in danger of breaking the lifelong commitment I had made to Him; a kind of emotional adultery. I went back to the Mission House and immediately made an appointment to go down to Hastings to see Mother Sarah Grace.

The night before I was due to go, there was an unexpected arrival at the front door of the Mission House. It was a wild, stormy night – gusty wind, rain lashing down in torrents, and for a moment I wondered whether or not I had really heard the bell ring. I decided to investigate and opened the door to find a soaking Marie-Louise, with her cape flapping and glasses covered in drops of rain. For a moment it felt like the scene from *The Princess and the Pea*, where the castle door swings open to find a random, drenched girl on the doorstep, claiming to be a real princess. I couldn't help but wonder if I put a pea underneath Marie-Louise's bed whether I would find out that she was a real Sister; and then I immediately asked God's forgiveness for such flippancy in light of what could only be an emergency. I hustled her in.

'Marie-Louise, what on earth are you doing here, on a night like tonight as well? Come in quickly.'

She started babbling.

'Oh, Sister Catherine Mary! Something dreadful has happened. I just couldn't stay. It was horrible. Just too, *too* horrible.'

'Oh, my dear! Let me fetch Sister Ruth and we must get you out of these wet clothes ...'

'No,'she put her hand on my arm. 'I'm not ready to speak to Sister Ruth yet. Can we just go to your room? I really would like to speak to you alone. Perhaps we don't need to let anyone know I'm here yet? Please?'

Well, this was all highly irregular and even though we had experienced nearly a whole decade of the Swinging Sixties' revolution, I automatically felt a pang of fear at doing something that would be considered 'irregular'. But Marie-Louise was beginning to sound a bit hysterical, so I said, 'OK then. Let's be quiet, though. Best not to frighten the horses, eh?'

She looked so alarmed, I had to put my arm round her. As we quietly went up the stairs together, I wondered what on earth had happened to break Marie-Louise's normal composure. The whole story came tumbling out as soon as we got to my room. I wanted to get her into dry clothes first, but she didn't seem to care.

'It was terrible! I was in the delivery room. And you know Mrs Coleman, from down March Street?'

'Oh, no! Don't tell me something has happened to her baby?'

She nodded, and started to sob.

'Dear Lord, no!' I said and crossed myself. Poor Margery Coleman had been trying to have a baby for years. She had had many miscarriages and an ectopic pregnancy. Infertility is a tragedy today, but in those days it held even more stigma. There was a huge premium for married women to have a family. It was still seen by most as the primary purpose for a woman if she hadn't given up on marriage in favour of a career like teaching or nursing. But now Margery finally seemed to be carrying a baby to term. It was an occasion of great joy to the whole Community and we had said prayers of thanks. Marie-Louise continued.

'Stupid junior doctor! Rubbish, totally rubbish! He was doing it all wrong. I knew he was doing it wrong, I just couldn't bring myself to say anything. I failed and now the poor baby is dead.'

'Oh, I am so sorry.'

I went over and put my arms round her. Both of us were crying now.

'He was breech and the doctor just wasn't doing anything. He botched the whole thing and I knew it. I could see what was going to happen. I said so, but he just wouldn't listen. I should have taken control.'

'How could you, though? How could you? It's not your fault; it isn't. You're only training. He's the doctor, it's his responsibility. Please don't blame yourself. I would have been the same.'

'You wouldn't! You would have said something. I know what you're like – you have courage.'

'No, not at your stage. That only comes with experience and you did speak.'

'Not loud enough.'

We cried together for a time and then I said, 'We can never know why some little souls are sent for such a short time on earth, but we know that God suffers with us in every tragedy we face in life.'

'You really believe that?'

I had to think for a moment. Then I said, 'I have to. Otherwise I couldn't do this job and witness the tragedies I have witnessed.'

Marie-Louise sat silently thinking and then she started crying again.

'Oh, it was dreadful – the scream that Margery made from every fibre of her being.'

I nodded. I remembered the Cyclops baby. There is a special terrible cry that mothers can make when they have lost their child and it haunts me.

'I had to take the baby to the mortuary. I wrapped him up, and you know the mortuary?'

I nodded. It was a short walk from the hospital, but it meant you had to go outside.

'It was pouring with rain and when I got there it was closed. I was stood outside, holding this dead baby in my arms. I knocked on the door and no one answered. So I just stood there in the rain and the baby was getting wet, and I was thinking, "This poor mite is getting soaked," and then I thought, "But he's dead, it doesn't matter," but it did. It was so disrespectful. Everything felt wrong. I stood there wondering what on earth God was playing at, may He forgive me.'

'He forgives you, Marie-Louise. He does. He understands our anger. We are allowed to be angry with Him and it is right to tell Him our anger. Put it in front of Him, tell Him everything you feel. You will find peace. It may take a long time but as long as you keep telling Him how you feel and laying it before Him, He will send you peace. You will be reconciled.'

'I hope you're right. At the moment it feels impossible. I feel like I can't go on.'

I held her some more, and then she drew back from me.

'And then, you know what? I kept banging on the door and eventually the mortician answered and said, "We're closed", and I was stood there with a dead baby in my arms.'

'Oh, no!'

'Yes. I said, "Look, I've got a dead baby here. What am I supposed to do? Are you just going to leave us out in the rain?" I shouted, I was so angry.'

'And?'

'Well, he let us in, but he was so rude. Unbelievable! I kept seeing poor Margery lying there and what she would think if she could see how her baby was being treated. The lack of humanity.'

I nodded.

I suggested we say a prayer together, for Margery and her baby boy, and also for Marie-Louise (and for the junior doctor and the mortician), and then I took Marie-Louise down to Sister Ruth.

The next day I boarded a train to the Mother House. All the way I was thinking about Marie-Louise and Margery Coleman; the horrific waste and the sheer agony. And somehow it put my own struggles with Father Ian into perspective. They seemed trivial, superficial and shabby, and most of all, selfish. I wondered whether this journey was necessary at all but as the buildings got smaller and sparser and suddenly the train was speeding through fields, I felt my spirits lighten. It was good to get out of London, to get some space.

I realised how much I needed a break. It was the beginning of March, and just at the cusp of spring, when some days it is definitely still winter and the next day it is definitely spring. As soon as I got to the Mother House I went for a walk. The bright spring sunshine was calling me out and to stay inside would feel like a reproach. Anyway, I needed to blow away my cobwebs, spring-clean and hang the freshly laundered white linen of my soul on the washing line and let it blow dry in the sun. As I walked along a footpath by the side of the fields the land was grey and barren, but when I looked closely at the trees they were full of buds just waiting to burst into life. There were catkins, an empty nest, bunny rabbits hopping with white tails bobbing, I saw crocuses and daffodils.

I felt the power of the turn of the earth. We get caught up in human stuff in the city, but out here all I could see was the overwhelming power of Nature and God's creation. Whatever we human beings were up to, summer was coming. Like ants, we scurry away oblivious to the fact that something much bigger is at work. A row of beautiful trees caught my eye, but then I noticed each one had a tremendous amount of ivy climbing up the trunks. While the branches were bare, the only thing that appeared to be living was the fecund ivy – lush green, thriving. I stopped and pondered it. It was beautiful, but wasn't it actually getting in the way? Didn't it need to be chopped back in order for the tree to thrive or even to survive? It was a parasite, a seductive one, but it was taking the goodness and shutting out the light. I spent a long time looking at this line of trees. 'Father Ian is my ivy,' I thought and I snapped off a piece of ivy to take back to my room and ponder further.

Sat in front of Mother Sarah Grace, I poured out my story; I held nothing back. I didn't know what to expect. I didn't know of anyone else whose chastity had been challenged during my time with the Community (or at least as far as I knew!). But Mother Sarah Grace sat impassive throughout, only raising an eyebrow when I confessed to being distracted by the back of Father Ian's neck during the Ecumenical Service. When I had finished she sat silently and closed her eyes. The clock ticked loudly in the corner. Time stretched. I could hear every sound: the birds in the garden, the distant clatter of plates, a door being slammed. After about five minutes she opened her eyes and started shuffling in the drawer of her desk.

'Sister Catherine Mary, thank you for coming to me with this. You did the right thing. I want to give you something.'

After a bit of rummaging she found what she wanted. She passed me a postcard of a painting. It was a depiction of Christ in the early dawn, standing at an overgrown door, about to knock. In his hand was a bright lamp.

'Do you know what this is?' she asked.

'Yes, Mother. It's "The Light of the World" by Holman Hunt. I saw it recently in St Paul's Cathedral – I found it rather powerful.'

'Indeed. And do you know what passage of scripture it was inspired by?'

'Yes. Some verse from Revelations, I think,

Behold, I stand at the door, and knock:
If anyone hear my voice, and open the door,
I will come in to him and sill sup with him, and he with me

'Well done, Sister. Exactly.'

'Exactly?'

'Christ is knocking at your door. You need to let him in.'

I was surprised and a little cross.

'But Mother, I *have* let him in! I couldn't have let him in further – I'm a nun!'

'It's not the habit you wear on the outside, Sister, it's what's going on inside that I'm concerned with.'

'But …' I tried to interrupt but she carried on.

'In our consecration to Christ we are always being called to a deeper understanding of ourselves, to deeper commitment and transformation. There will be temptations but it is what you do with them that matters. Now what you have to do in this case is to do exactly what any spouse should do when tempted to break their vows, and that is step away from the temptation and fill the gap by spending more time getting closer and more intimate with the person they married – which, in your case, is God.' She made a nod in the direction of my wedding ring.

'I would suggest you spend the day here in prayer then go back refreshed and renewed to face the situation. I would also suggest that you pray about your future, asking for discernment for your way forward in the religious life and the development of your ministry as a midwife.'

I sat in silence and then I had a small epiphany: a picture of Marie-Louise came into my head.

'Mother, I think I would like to train to be a midwife tutor. I would like to teach.'

Mother Sarah Grace paused and looked at me.

'I think that is an excellent idea, Sister. While you are here I shall start making enquiries and see what can be done. In the meantime, keep the postcard and meditate on it. Listen for Christ knocking; let him come further into your life.'

I left her study and felt an enormous, tearful sense of relief and gratitude. Everything suddenly made sense and I felt like I had come home. In my room I went down on my knees in front of the postcard with the ivy laid at its feet and thanked God for this moment of insight. I didn't want any midwife to go through what Marie-Louise had just been through and if I could prevent just one baby from losing its life in the way that Margery Coleman's baby had lost his life, then any personal sacrifice would be worth it. I had been working in midwifery for five years and now I wanted to teach everything I knew about being a midwife, to make sure midwives had the confidence to speak up; that women were not 'done unto' but empowered to bring their babies safely into the world. It all made sense. I also took another long look at the ivy and realised that the ivy was not so much Father

Ian as the loneliness I had felt since Cecilia had gone. My relationship with Father Ian was a symptom, not a cause.

A few weeks later back in Poplar, I was summoned to the telephone and Mother Sarah Grace informed me that a place had been found for me to return to the London Lying-In Hospital in preparation for applying to train as a midwife tutor at the Midwifery Training School in Kingston. This all felt right and I was excited; whatever madness I had been seized with had disappeared in a puff of smoke, the daft fog had cleared and the whole landscape looked different. Indeed, the very thought of seeing Father Ian made me feel slightly sick.

When I think of life as a journey, as lots of people do, I often wonder whether it is a maze or a labyrinth. The difference between a maze and a labyrinth is that mazes have dead ends and false paths whereas labyrinths only have one path and as long as you put one foot in front of the other you will reach the centre, even if sometimes, geographically, you have to go further away first. Sometimes my life has seemed like a maze – my infatuation with Father Ian could, in some ways, be seen as a classic false path to a dead end. And yet if it hadn't been for Father Ian, I doubt that I would ever have become a midwife tutor.

For the next 18 months I found myself back as a student, training. I enjoyed it immensely and felt that I really was in the right place, doing the right thing. However, towards the end of 1969 when I had only three months still to do and I was really looking forward to qualifying and starting teaching, I was suddenly faced with a change of direction that felt as if I had been wrenched out of the maze by a bulldozer or suddenly had a Minotaur blocking the path of the labyrinth.

Alarm bells started to ring as soon as the letter arrived from Mother Sarah Grace, asking me to go to Hastings to attend a meeting with the Bishop of Malawi. Now what would he be wanting? My instincts told me nothing good. So I took myself off at the weekend up to London to visit the Nursing and Midwifery Show at Earls Court. Not that I particularly wanted to go, but I knew Sister Alice would be there. I scoured the busy arena and it wasn't long before I said to myself, 'Hyacinth, darling'. In the distance was the happy bright blue of a habit from the Community of St John the Divine. I pushed my way through the crowds and tapped the shoulder of my old teacher and mentor, Sister Alice. She turned round, her face broke into a broad grin and she gave me a warm hug as I said, 'Sister Alice, I'm so glad I have found you! You are just the person I need to see.'

'Well, Sister Catherine Mary, this is an unexpected and blessed pleasure!'

'Come and have a cup of tea with me straight away. There's something I want to show you.'

As we each sat with a cup of strong tea and a rock cake, I produced Mother Sarah Grace's request for attendance at a meeting with the Bishop of Malawi.

'Well, what do you think?' I asked Sister Alice.

'What is there to think?'

'Well, don't you think it's suspicious?'

'No. Why?'

'Well, what's behind it? What does he want? I don't like the sound of it.'

'Don't be ridiculous! There's nothing behind it. He just wants to visit the Community. Honestly, Sister Catherine Mary, you always did have an overactive imagination and a tendency to the dramatic.' She rolled her eyes, tutted in mock disgust and then changed the subject to discuss the arrival of the new curate at All Saints Church.

So I sat on my suspicions, went back to college and then on the allotted day took the train to Hastings to meet the Bishop. On arrival, I found all the Sisters had been summoned. I looked around and tried to make some sort of sense of what we were all doing there. Sister Alice had come after all and with her was Marie-Louise. Interesting. Marie-Louise had overcome the trauma of Mrs Coleman's baby's death and been persuaded by Sister Ruth to go back and complete her training at the hospital, and then Part Two in the district, and now she was a fully qualified midwife. In fact, she had taken my place working in Poplar. I could understand Sister Alice's presence as a senior midwife and member of the Community, but why would Marie-Louise have been brought all the way down here? All the nerves in my body started to jangle.

The Bishop of Malawi was a loud, jolly, charismatic man. For three hours he talked to us and kept us enthralled (in a rather horrified way). He described a desperate situation. In Malawi, in 1969 there were hardly any trained midwives or hospitals with dedicated maternity units. Proper antenatal and post-natal care were limited. Death rates for both mothers and babies were equivalent to mid-Victorian England. So many of these deaths, and the poverty and heartbreak they brought, could have been avoided with just some basic medical care. There was a little hospital called St Anne's in a place called Nkhotakota, which had been run by Christian missionaries for many decades. Now the Bishop had come to England to ask if the Community of St John's could take it over, and expand it. He wanted us to set up a proper maternity unit and start a midwifery training school, which could eventually be taken over by the government and set the template for an expansion of maternity services across the whole of Malawi. It would ensure proper care would be available to women not just in the towns, but also in the more rural areas of the country. He thought that this would take five years.

At the end of his speech Mother Sarah Grace thanked him, and said that the Community would think and pray about his request and get back to him. I knew it – I had known it all along.

In the following weeks the Sisters prayed and consulted, and I was summoned back to speak to Mother Sarah Grace.

'Sister Catherine Mary, you know we have been asked to take over the hospital of St Anne's in Malawi. After much prayer we have decided to answer this call. This means we need to send three Sisters over to Malawi and we would like one of those to be you. Indeed, we would like you to be in charge of the hospital.'

I knew it. But every nerve in my body didn't just jangle, it screamed 'No!' I tried to keep calm.

'Mother, I am just about to complete my training to be a midwife tutor. Everything has led me here; everything I have ever done. This is my path and this is my calling; I am sure of this. Everything is telling me I am not supposed to leave this path. Not at this time. Not when I am so close to reaching my God-given destination.'

'Sister Catherine Mary, none of us should ever presume to know our destination. God has called you for whatever reason to a greater purpose.'

'No. I'm not disagreeing with the purpose. It's a good and noble purpose but it's not mine. Why don't you send someone else?'

'There is no one else. Everyone else is committed, you are relatively free. You will have finished your studies in a few months and then you will be at liberty. You can resume your vocation as a midwife tutor when you get back. This is a much greater responsibility and opportunity for you. You will be in charge not just of setting up a school for midwives, but developing the whole maternity hospital.'

My head ached, I felt sick; it was too much.

'I don't want to do it. I want to be a midwife tutor here and sending me there – well, it's too much responsibility.'

'Well, you may not want to but you are being called. Go away and pray about it. Ask the Lord's opinion. You might be surprised by the answer. You have three weeks and then you will have to give the Chapter your decision.'

'Yes, Mother.' I bowed my head and sighed.

As I rose to leave, I realised there was another important question I hadn't asked.

'Mother, who else is being asked to go?'

'Sister Belinda has got experience of missionary work, but is now too advanced in years to take on the responsibility of the hospital so we have asked her to consider going to look after the House where you shall live. Also, Marie-Louise has been asked to accompany you and be your assistant.'

I nodded. There was method in their madness and I knew straight away, she was right: there was no one else free to take charge. But still I did not want to do it.

I spent the next few weeks in prayer but as sometimes happens when you really want Him to speak, God was silent. I had a horrible feeling He was silent because I wasn't letting him get a word in edgeways; I didn't want to hear what He had to say. So when I made the journey to the Chapter meeting I still didn't know what answer I was going to give to the Community. Well, I knew what answer I wanted to give – a loud 'No' – but I didn't know whether I would be brave enough to stand there and face the Community and let the word out of my mouth.

Once again I found myself standing in front of the semi-circle of my peers, Mother Sarah Grace in central position.

'Sister Catherine Mary, will you accept this mission and go to Malawi and run St Anne's Hospital?'

I opened my mouth to say no but 'yes' came out, and in front of me the Sisters' faces broke into smiles. I have no idea how it happened. Perhaps the most obvious explanation is the Holy Spirit momentarily leapt in and took over my faculties of speech – that's how it felt, anyway. But once the word was out of my mouth there was no going back. The meeting quickly moved on to practicalities and I was left thinking, 'Hang on, can we just roll back and I'll answer that again?' In the weeks that followed I kept on plucking up courage to go and tell the Reverend Mother that I'd changed my mind, but I'd get to her door and my hand couldn't physically reach up to knock. In the end I just had to accept, that whatever I felt about it, it was not just the Sisters but God Himself who wanted me to go.

So as the boat to Cape Town sailed out of Southampton harbour and we left the coast of England behind (the first time, in fact, I had ever left the coast of my native land), the wind played havoc with my headdress and the tears (of grief, I think) rolled unchecked down my cheeks. A favourite passage from Corinthian which I adapted, came into my head,

When I was a child, I spoke like a child, I thought like a child, I reasoned like a child. When I became a man, I gave up childish ways. For now we see through a glass darkly; but then face to face. Now I know in part; then I shall know fully, even as I have been fully known. So now faith, hope, and love abide, these three; but the greatest of these is love.

I never saw Father Ian again. Soon after I had started training at Kingston I had received a letter from him, telling me he had been transferred to a new parish at the other end of the country. We continued to write to each other intermittently for years. But it was interesting: he never did marry and, of course, neither did I.

CHAPTER TEN

THE TROUBLE WITH PARADISE

The first year in Malawi I was full of enthusiasm; the second year I started to get tired; the third year I was on my knees, and the fourth year I could hardly put one foot in front of the other. You didn't have to be a prophet to have predicted this – the clues were there right from the start. On my first weekend in Nkhotakota, I went for a little walk to get my bearings. I found myself around the back of the little missionary church, in a graveyard. It was poorly tended, with gravestones sticking through the long grass just enough to be able to make out the names on them:

Lillian Smith RIP 1900–1930

Poor Lillian! Thirty years old, two years younger than me. I wondered what had happened to her.

Then I looked at the gravestone next to her:

Paul Whetstone RIP 1911–1935

Twenty-four years old. With a sense of mounting panic, I started scanning the rest of the headstones. I found several names of early missionaries, and not one living beyond the age of 35. There were no clues as to how they had died, but it didn't look good.

I walked over to Lake Malawi; it stretched over the horizon like a sea – a long thin strip of water over 350 miles long, the ninth-largest lake in the world. Nk'otakota was one of the 60 towns and villages that had grown up along its banks, and I could see in the distance the mud huts of the next village. The water twinkled blue in the early morning sunshine and there were men fishing in small boats.

I remembered reading in an encyclopedia borrowed from the library in the Mother House that Lake Malawi had more species of fish than any other freshwater lake in the world. Steamboats went backwards and forwards, some probably off to Mozambique on the other side. They reminded me of the film *The African Queen*, which I had seen as a teenager. Then, Africa seemed impossibly exotic and remote. Yet here I was like some 1970s Katharine Hepburn. No sign of a Humphrey Bogart to corrupt my missionary work, though, I chuckled to myself.

Down near the beach an impromptu bazaar had appeared. Large pieces of driftwood had been used to set up stalls of fruit and colourful materials. Children were playing while women haggled. The smell of Africa –

damp, rich earth mixed with tropical flowers like hibiscus and frangipani – overpowered me.

How could somewhere so close to Paradise hide such mortal sickness?

The answer was there in front of me – diarrhoea, vomiting and malaria were rife among the people. As I looked at the tiny waves whipped up by the gentle breeze, I remembered why none of the children were actually in the water. Beneath the pretty blue lurked bilharzia, parasitic worms that, while rarely fatal, result in lifelong illness and all sorts of damage to your internal organs. There was danger in paradise, as if the more beautiful the landscape, the more deadly it could be. In a way that was exactly the reason why God had sent us here, but at what cost? It seemed that others who had come before us, doing His work, had paid the ultimate price.

Despite this nagging fear lurking at the back of my consciousness, it was amazing how quickly I left smoggy, cold London behind and became acclimatised to my hot, exotic new home.

It had started on the boat over. Sister Rachel had made us some new habits that were more appropriate for tropical Africa. And gosh, how ridiculously exciting that was – a new outfit for the first time in years! We were allowed to have a say in the design and we decided on pale blue habits with short sleeves and skirts ending just below the knee, and shorter, lighter white headdresses. (Of course our crosses of St John and girdles were eternal.)

As we sailed over the equator and the weather heated up, we abandoned heavy old home clothes and put on our new habits. One day, as we sat outside on stripy deckchairs, becalmed and sweltering in the South Atlantic Ocean, Sister Marie-Louise exclaimed, 'Lord preserve us! Would it really matter if we took off the undercap?'

Sister Belinda and I looked at each other.

'No, no, I don't think it would – not if we all do it. Shall we?' I asked.

'I'm game,' Sister Belinda said. So we retreated to our rooms and emerged like butterflies from a chrysalis, lighter and transformed, never to put them on again.

The transformation continued once we got off the ship at Cape Town and started our ten-day train journey north across Africa to Malawi. I gazed out of the window at landscapes that seemed to have come straight out of a picture book – an idea that wasn't helped by reading the whole of *The Lord of the Rings*. It had just come out and looked reassuringly thick, the kind of book that you might be able to read several times, which considering I was a bit like a guest on *Desert Island Discs* who can only take one book besides the Bible and the complete works of Shakespeare (books would be few and far between in Malawi and I didn't have much room in my suitcase), Tolkien it was. And although it's not supposed to be religious, it is about good versus evil, and I could see Christ in there, so it proved to be a good choice. But which seemed more unreal, the book or the view from the window? I wasn't sure.

When we arrived in Malawi, the jolly Bishop put us up in his colonial house for a few days while we recovered from the journey, and then we set off on a long jeep ride deep into the centre of the country, to our final destination – the small clusters of settlements known as Nkhotakota.

Our little patch in Nkhotakota was like an African version of the square back in Poplar. The hub of the community was a large quadrangle, with an enormous tree at its centre. On the one side was the missionary church, with the graveyard behind; at right-angles to it was a primary school and opposite this was the hospital. Down a dirt track was another square with more buildings – houses for the various volunteers and missionaries, and our new home, which we would rename St John's House. Again, in the middle was a large tree that had apparently been planted by David Livingstone in 1859, when he stayed there resting on his journey to find the source of the River Nile. Everywhere there were flowers and mango trees. At first glance it really was quite beautiful.

However, on closer inspection it became clear what we were up against. The new St John's House had only the most basic furniture. Luckily, we had been warned and we came with trunks full of linen and cutlery. The roof was made of corrugated iron and leaked. One night there was a terrific downpour and I dreamt I was being rained upon. I woke to find a trickle of drips pouring onto my forehead. Marie-Louise was sleeping in a little bed on the other side of the room and seemed to be dry, so I pushed my bed across the room next to hers. But as the rain continued, we both started to get splashed.

'Botheration! This is no good,' I said. 'Let's go and see if we can slip in with Sister Belinda.'

So we scurried down the corridor and opened the door to Sister Belinda's room, only to find her sitting bolt upright in bed, holding an umbrella over her head! Luckily, there was an easy solution which involved offering a small amount of pocket money to some of the local lads, who were only too happy to spend a day on our roof.

The hospital itself was a greater worry: the wards were made up of tiny beds or mats placed tightly next to each other on the floor, so that there was barely any room for us to get between them. It had space for 60 patients, but there were always more than 100 women needing treatment. During the day it was so hot (generally over 100°F) that the verandah was full of heavily pregnant women sitting or lying, all trying desperately to keep cool.

There was only one labour ward, which consisted of four walls and two iron beds with rubber mats. There were some bowls and disinfectant in a kidney dish, a pair of forceps and some scissors and clamps; the only light was a Tilley lamp. It had to be held in the right position, otherwise we would have had to deliver babies in the middle of the night in total darkness (and the African night could be *very* dark). This meant that there always needed to be two of us up, one to cross-match the blood and the other to be down at the business end.

It has to be said that this was not necessarily a bad thing; generally the mothers who arrived at the hospital were those who needed emergency care. No matter how experienced, I always found it helpful to have a second opinion and support if things went wrong. And they did go wrong. To my horror we did lose mothers and babies from the start, women and children who would not have died in the East End of London, because we just didn't have the equipment or the expertise to deal with some of the extreme emergencies we faced.

The most obvious problem was that we didn't have an operating theatre. If an emergency Caesarean was needed, the mother would have to be transported at great risk to the main hospital, which was a ten-minute drive. But we only had one method of getting them there, which was the old Land Rover, and if that was already off at the hospital, or on an errand, or even acting as a mobile clinic going round the local villages, we would face an agonising wait.

We had two men helping us in the house – Anton, who cleaned and drove the Land Rover, and Henry, who cooked. Jobs were scarce in Malawi, so we were encouraged to employ local men with families who badly needed a steady income. Anton and Henry were both devout Christians, with lots of mouths depending on them to be fed, so they were immensely grateful for the full-time, secure jobs we gave them. Nothing was ever too much trouble.

Henry was smaller, more inscrutable and intense. Anton, on the other hand, was tall, lanky and funny. He became my right-hand man. Driving me from emergency to emergency, singing hymns (sometimes changing the words), giving a running commentary and gently teasing me (he insisted on calling me 'Reverend Mama'). Meanwhile in the hospital we had the help of a Dutch doctor who regularly visited and a rich American volunteer called Eloise. Two years before she had come out for a short eight-week placement, but ended up staying for eight months, then went home and then came back indefinitely with her baby grand piano. Every evening she used to play it with the french windows open and sometimes we would go and sit on the grass in the quad and listen. I used to watch Sister Belinda (the former concert pianist) listening impassively and wonder if it was torture for her. One day, I said to her, 'Go on, why don't you ask Eloise if you can have a go? I'm sure she'd be delighted.'

I regretted it immediately. Sister Belinda looked hurt and vigorously shook her head.

'That was my old life. It has no place with me now.'

I wanted to argue with her. Why on earth not? Just because we have started a new life, does that mean we have to reject everything of the old, even the most creative, positive bits? But I sensed at that moment it was more important to respect Sister Belinda's approach to her vocation, so I remained silent.

On my first day I was bewildered by the sheer mass of people and weight of things that needed to be done. There was an extraordinary line of women and young children winding all the way out of the hospital and up the road, with more coming and joining from all directions. They didn't seem to be pregnant. I asked one of the nurses what was going on.

'Oh, that's the vaccination clinic,' she said.

'Vaccinations? But these children are quite old, some of them look about five.'

'Well, we're a maternity hospital.'

'Yes, exactly. What are these people doing here, they don't look pregnant?'

'Well, part of the job of the maternity hospital is to look after the health of the babies until they are five.'

'Hang on, in England a baby is a baby until about the age of one year and then they become a child! And anyway, a baby is only the responsibility of the maternity hospital until they are six weeks old and then they are handed into the care of the health visitor.'

The nurse shrugged.

'In Malawi, maternity hospitals look after the child until they are five.'

That was a bit of a shock. It meant we were responsible for the health of all the children in the area until the age of five – a huge job for any unit, but especially in an area where so many children were vulnerable to disease and malnutrition. 'I will not be scared, I will not be scared,' I repeated over and over to myself, and I made a mental note to send off as soon as possible for a book on basic paediatrics from the London School of Hygiene & Tropical Medicine.

The responsibility of being in charge of all this was feeling a bit overwhelming. But I decided the best place to start was to make an inventory of the equipment in the hospital, if only to see what was missing. I found myself weeping as I examined the medieval-looking forceps; I was filled with the admiration for the missionaries we had replaced, having to work under such conditions. As I was wiping away my tears, a woman came running in and tugged on my sleeve.

'Uko.'

'Uko?' I repeated.

She nodded and said again in Chichewa, 'Uko.'

I turned to our volunteer, Eloise.

'What does she mean?'

'Uko, over there.'

'Over there?'

'Yes, it's what they say when someone is trying to get here and has collapsed. We call it the "Failed to walk" phenomenon.'

'Dear God!'

'Well, they end up having to walk miles. There aren't any cars out in the villages, you know.'

'Well, of course, but what am I supposed to do about it?'

'You send someone out in the Land Rover to find them and bring them in.'

'OK.'

I turned to the woman and said: 'Uko, where?'

She nodded and pointed in the general direction of the hospital door. Eloise laughed.

'That's the best you're going to get, Sister! They don't do things like maps or directions.'

'Dear God!' I exclaimed again, 'How on earth does anyone ever survive here?'

'Well, they do, Sister, they generally do. You're just going to have to relax, go into Malawi gear and up your praying.'

I studied Eloise carefully and decided I liked the cut of her jib.

'OK. Eloise, would you be kind enough to take this lady and go and find Anton – I think he's in the house. See if he can drive around with her and locate her friend and bring her in.'

'Righty-ho, Sister.'

Half an hour later Anton returned with a labouring, but grinning lady in bright clothes. And that's what struck me going round the wards – the stoicism of the women. They were calm and uncomplaining despite the heat and lack of facilities, always terribly respectful and grateful. During the day I witnessed five babies being born, and rarely had I been present at such quiet births. Were they experiencing less pain? It's impossible to know, but my hunch is that, having grown up without a pot of painkillers ready to hand, they were just better at dealing with it.

I also felt there might be something psychologically deeper going on. They were deeply religious, with a depth of faith that would put most of our woolly Anglican churchgoers to shame. It was humbling. But also during our first month, the other Sisters and I were taken to see a traditional ceremony for a first time mother-to-be. I suppose it was the Malawi equivalent of an antenatal class that extended into the labour itself. It took place in a secret location outside the village. The only people allowed to be present were women who already had children (they made an exception for us on the grounds that we were 'medical staff').

The women sat in a circle with the new mother at the end of her pregnancy, freshly washed, in the middle. Her mother then came and danced for her, wearing a corn on a cob tied around her middle. The corn represented the baby. She sang a song, which she had composed herself, where she went through every stage of childbirth in great detail so the new mother would know exactly what to expect. It was very moving. It was then explained to me that she would be taken back into the hut where she would give birth, surrounded by the mothers of the village. The men would wait outside, and when the baby had been born it would be washed and the mother washed and dressed, and brought out and presented to the village. There would then be great rejoicing, with the traditional noise made with fingers waggling in their mouths. Somehow it seemed to me that the Malawi women were as well prepared by this ritual as British women are by their antenatal classes.

I was still struggling with the enormity of the responsibility until I had a bit of an epiphany in my second week. One afternoon the local Mothers Union came to sing and dance for us. They stood under the big tree in the centre of the quad, while the patients shuffled or even crawled on to the verandah, and started to sing low gospel songs, swaying, clapping and laughing. Everyone who could joined in. Before I knew it, I found myself shifting my weight from one foot to the other and clapping.

Sister Marie-Louise stuck her head out of a window and raised her eyebrows at me. I didn't care – I was the boss now. This was a thought that hadn't struck me before, and I suddenly felt terribly liberated. Yes, I had huge new responsibilities but with them came a new freedom. My life as a nurse and a midwife, and as a Sister, had been extremely ordered. I had been in institutions for a long time, and I'd had a place in a strict hierarchy (usually somewhere towards the bottom). The standards of procedure, order and cleanliness demanded by both my profession and my calling back in England were very ingrained. They were the canvas and foundation upon which I had worked, and had seemed an absolute prerequisite for any sort of success. Now I realised these standards would have to be left back in England and I would need to learn a new flexibility and resourcefulness.

After supper I took a long walk outside. The clarity of the sky was overwhelming. The stars were so bright and close I felt like impersonating Henny Penny and running for cover to stop them dropping on my head. Fireflies danced around me. I couldn't help but fancy them little Tinker Bell fairies – 'Sprinkle your dust on me and take me to Peter,' I said – then I remembered myself and said a much more serious prayer: 'Dear Lord, thank you for bringing me here and letting me witness such a different, amazing piece of Your creation.'

And as I spoke, in the distance there were flashes of forked lightning, igniting the sky. I wondered where all my resistance to this adventure had gone; I seemed to have left it behind at Southampton docks. I felt terribly liberated and energised. Eloise's words about getting into Malawi gear came to mind. My head was racing with plans for the hospital. The scale of the task might be overwhelming but if I approached it with the attitude that I could never make it into a mini London Lying-In Hospital, but instead every little improvement I made was a step in the right direction, that would justify my presence here, and I would have done my job.

I was drawn towards the lake and walked along the shore. I could see the twinkling lanterns of the fishing boats. When David Livingstone had been here he had called it the Lake of Stars because of these twinkling lanterns. A hundred years later, so little had changed. Then I went back and sat on the little bench under the big tree in the middle of the quad as the lightning flashed around me, and the old familiar prayer of St Francis of Assisi came to mind:

> *God grant me the serenity to accept the things I*
> *   cannot change,*
> *The courage to change the things I can,*
> *And the wisdom to know the difference.*

Then I got a little notebook out of my pocket and started to make a list of all the things I wanted to do.

The next day I grabbed Marie-Louise and Anton, and we took a trip into the nearest town. We bought every pot of paint and paintbrush we could lay our hands on and then, with bribes of pennies, we hired some of the local young men and emptied the hospital, room by room. We took out the beds, ward by ward, and laid them out in the sun to air while we swept the floors thoroughly. Our patients lay under the big tree while the children repainted the rooms in cheery colours – red, yellow, green and blue. (And Anton singing 'Red and yellow and pink and green', or 'Dear Lord and Father of mankind, Forgive our Foolish Green, repaint us all in purer mind, in purer lives thy service find', or 'Paint then wherever you may be, I am the Lord of the Paint said He', or any ridiculous variation he could think of.)

We then put health charts on the walls. Not that we needed them, but just to give the place the feeling of being professional.

Right from the start I knew that my most important task was to set up the midwifery school. Once I had installed a proper training programme, there would be a constant stream of qualified professionals who could then go out and spread their expertise across Malawi. First of all we had to build classrooms, a library and accommodation. We were asked to take 20 students on a two-year course. During that time they would have lessons with Marie-Louise, Belinda and me, and have practical experience working with us out on the ward (which was probably the most useful bit).

For reasons I never quite understood, the Dutch government had given the money for the new buildings before we came, so we were able to start work straight away. For our first six months in Nkhotakota, the quad was a building site. I didn't know anything about building to begin with, but by the end I thought if ever I was defrocked, I could get a job working on a construction site. Men were forever running into the hospital, asking, 'Excuse me, Mama, sorry Mama, shall we dig the trench now?'

I didn't know, but actually most of the enquiries just seemed to be a matter of common sense, so I guessed the answers and the buildings got built. Of course we did have a Master of Works, but he was often busy off-site. And indeed he *had* been busy. One day he and a young

English lady volunteer walked into the kitchen, hand in hand, and announced their engagement.

We had a wonderful wedding in the church; I loved being in there. The priest's vestments and the altar furnishings were ancient and elaborately embroidered. They must have been brought over 100 years ago by the original missionaries, and for me they were a tangible link with our missionary past. The Malawians were so exuberant, the most wonderful uninhibited singers, making up beautiful harmonies as they went along, usually singing our traditional hymns in their own Chichewa language. Especially for the wedding, someone found an old pedal organ and the church was filled with all the locals who crowded in to see what a traditional Western wedding would look like. I did shed a tear – it was a wonderful day. But as I watched them pack up and the young volunteer and her Master of Works disappear up the dirt track to start a new life elsewhere, suddenly I felt a bit left behind.

However, this didn't last for long, although it took an unexpected accident to set me back on the path. First, I must point out that food played a very important part in the religious life. When so many avenues are closed to you, a bit like being a prisoner or a patient in hospital, food is eagerly anticipated and relished.

It's not difficult to fulfill the Grace, 'For what we are about to receive, May the Lord make us truly thankful'. We generally were; except in Malawi. My goodness, the food was monotonous! With transport links practically non-existent, we were totally reliant on what the local earth could provide. So, breakfast every day was fruit, often the kind of fruit you can't get in many supermarkets even today – pawpaws, guavas, passion fruit and granadillas. Lunch would be maize flour with groundnuts and dinner was fish straight from the lake. It sounds appealing but I hated it. Boiled, steamed, baked or fried, cooked every which way, but always fish. I longed for meat.

Once a month we would take turns to get into the Land Rover with Anton and drive the 75 miles to Lilongwe with a shopping list. This meant when we got back there would be a few days of fresh meat for everyone. It was an eagerly anticipated event.

A couple of months after the wedding I went off with Anton to do the shopping, but on the way back, on a dusty windy road in the searing heat, the car broke down. We spent five hours trying to start it. I began to feel a bit panicky but Anton made me laugh, 'Don't worry, Reverend Mama. It'll be OK – the Lord will save us.'

Then he started to sing loudly in his rich, low voice,

She who would valiant be 'gainst all disaster,
Let her in constancy follow the Master.
There's no discouragement shall make her once relent
Her first avowed intent, to be a pilgrim.

Now when I find myself in a tricky situation, I start singing Anton's feminist version of the old crusading hymn.

Well, as he had predicted, help did eventually come in the form of a lorry. The driver got out a rope and started towing us along the road. But we hadn't gone very far when there was an almighty explosion. The Land Rover's tyre burst, sending us spinning off the road and down a slope, saved only by the rope holding us to the lorry. Somehow we managed to get ourselves out and then tow the car back onto the road, change the wheel and get home. But more drama followed when I realised I had left all the food by the side of the road. I was devastated. We did often long for our usual Western food, and that food parcel with its fresh meat was so important to the spirits of the Community, so I felt as if I had let them all down. However, the next day a huge food parcel arrived from home, and then someone left ten eggs on our doorstep, and then someone else gave us the gift of a chicken for the safe delivery of his daughter. Actually, in the end we didn't lack for anything and I was put in mind of a passage from the scriptures:

> *Consider the lilies how they grow; they toil not, they spin not; and yet I say unto you, that Solomon in all his glory was not arrayed like one of these.*

'Don't worry, the Lord will provide,' I told myself. But I wondered whether He was doing more than that when a few days later we finally got the Land Rover to a garage. The mechanic turned the key in the ignition and the car started straight away. He could find nothing wrong with it.

'Lord be praised!' Anton said. 'If the car hadn't broken down, then we would have been driving when the tyre burst, and we would have spun off the road, down the slope and could have been killed. It's a miracle. Thank you, gracious Lord.'

The mechanic nodded and crossed himself. I wasn't entirely convinced – the car might not have spun completely off the road, we might not have been on the edge of a slope at the time, and we might not have been killed. But then again, here I was alive, and for what purpose? It did feel like a message.

And this feeling grew as I became more confident in my midwifery work at the hospital. Before we came out, Sisters Belinda and Marie-Louise and I discussed that we would probably have to do procedures that only doctors were allowed to do in England. As soon as I arrived, I realised I would have to perform ventouse deliveries. This is where a vacuum device is placed on the head of the baby to assist birth when the mother is having difficulty pushing the baby out herself. We did sometimes have a doctor visit the hospital but he was more often than not somewhere else. Very soon I was facing a situation when I had to deliver a baby myself with the ventouse. I was nervous but as I told myself, I had witnessed this procedure many times before and I was very clear what had to be done, and if a doctor could do it, then why shouldn't I be able to do so?

A young mother was in the hospital with her second baby. I could feel that the birth canal was adequate and the baby was importantly in the correct position, but she had been labouring for a long time and was exhausted, and the baby was not progressing. So I placed the suction cap on the head of the baby and as she had a contraction, I gently pulled. Within several contractions the baby was delivered. It was a wonderful feeling (and a huge relief) that I could do it. After that I regularly used the ventouse. Sometimes it only took a few minutes, sometimes up to half an hour (particularly if it was a first baby), but it usually worked.

Very occasionally the birth canal was just too small to allow a normal delivery and a small cut had to be made through the back of the symphysis pubis (the joint that unites the public bones), at the front of the pelvis to enlarge the birth canal. Delivery could often then take place with a ventouse. This procedure is never done now in developed countries, you would just perform a Caesarean section. But in developing countries like Malawi, where the option to have a Caesarean isn't necessarily there, they still sometimes have to be performed. Afterwards the mother's pelvis would be a bit wobbly, so I had a very useful leather case strap, which I used to place round, her pelvis to hold it up securely while she healed.

And then I faced a situation that was always going to happen – a mother who had a fully obstructed labour and needed a Caesarean to save her life. We diagnosed that she was obstructed, we knew she needed a Caesarean section and we also knew that the doctor was stuck behind flood water, some 80 miles away. I watched her for hours, labouring in great pain, and it was obvious that unless something was done her uterus was liable to rupture and she would likely die.

'She's going to die, Dear God, tell me what to do,' I prayed.

I watched and prayed in agony as the woman's contractions grew more desperate and she got weaker. There was nothing I could do – or was there? Unbeknown to me the staff had already started preparing one of the rooms as an operating theatre. Suddenly I knew: this woman was going to die, for sure. But I had a choice – I should try to help her myself and if she died, well at least I had tried; it had got to the point where I felt there was nothing to lose. I asked for a room to be prepared, and then they told they'd already done it.

I've never seen a woman moved into theatre so quickly but even as we got her onto the table, her uterus ruptured. However, it was possible to remove the baby, who had already died, and the placenta then sew her up and repair the rupture. To my utter amazement she did indeed survive. When the doctor eventually arrived he said, 'I don't suppose you sterilised her at the same time, did you?'

'No, I jolly well didn't!' I said, probably a bit abruptly.

That night I thanked God for giving me the courage to act. A baby had died, but a woman lived to be able to return to her village and her family. It didn't take long working in the hospital to feel that I was doing something really important, and I no longer felt left behind by the departure of the Master of Works and the volunteer, but blessed.

Towards the end of our first year in Malawi, this feeling was reinforced when I hosted the grand opening of the new Midwifery Training School. The Dutch Ambassador was coming especially to see where their government's money had been spent and I had to make a speech. I was determined to make some of it in Chichewa, as well as in English, so everyone could understand.

We decided to get the Ambassador to plant a tree to commemorate the occasion. The building work had mainly been done with the help of non-violent prisoners, who came in trucks every day from the local jail. On the morning of the ceremony I asked one of them to dig a hole outside the Midwifery School to plant the tree in. Rather inconveniently, the labour ward suddenly got very busy, so I was otherwise engaged when one of the student midwives came running in: 'Mama, you come. Man, dig big hole up to shoulders.'

I went running out to find the prisoner had dug a hole big enough to bury himself in standing up. Seeing as the tree was only a tiny sapling it seemed a bit like overkill.

The opening ceremony was a joyful occasion. I made a short speech to the accompanying dignitaries in Chichewa. By then we had recruited 20 student midwives. They were mainly qualified nurses who wanted to continue their training to get midwifery skills as well, and I have to say I generally found these nurses the best to work with because they had a basic foundation on which to build. I decided that we should alternate days between working in English and then working in Chichewa, so there was a feeling of equality in the hospital and we all learned from each other.

Our teaching facilities were terribly basic – a blackboard and a piece of chalk and one textbook – Margaret Myles' old standard text on midwifery. It helped a bit – it did have pictures – but the level of English was above most of the students' capabilities and it was too technical. We also didn't have the equipment that was in the book, so it wasn't appropriate for the students to rely on. But still, the students were generally very dedicated. We gave them beautiful blue uniforms made by Sister Belinda, which they loved and kept immaculate. They had different coloured belts according to what stage they were at.

It was a great opportunity for the students: at the end of their course they would sit national exams, which would give them a qualification they could take to other places, and they were proud to be with us. I was particularly fond of Molly, who arrived as a trained nurse and stayed with us after she qualified, working her way up to become a staff midwife. She was a lovely, happy, reliable girl and it gave me great pleasure to see her grow in confidence and rely increasingly on her own judgement.

During my time in Malawi a phrase of my mother's kept coming to mind – 'necessity is the mother of invention'. For example, when a mother died and the baby lived (as unfortunately still occasionally happened), the student midwives would have to look after the child until the baby's family was located in the surrounding countryside and they had made a decision which of the extended family members would take responsibility for the baby. Sometimes this would take a long time. One little girl stayed with us for six months. Her family seemed in no hurry to come down to the hospital and claim her. It proved no problem, she lived permanently strapped to whichever student midwife was most free on the day, and was a very useful addition in our baby skills classes. She got a lot of nappy changes and baths. Occasionally she slept in my room when she was ill, but as I was usually up each night delivering babies, I didn't get to know her that well. When she was finally collected, there was much weeping from the students.

As it turned out I was right to have been intimidated by our responsibility for the care of the under-fives. Between 800 and 1,000 children had to be seen every year as part of the government's health and vaccination programme. Generally, about seven in every ten children who arrived at the clinic were malnourished. The most severe cases had to go into the hospital, but for the others we converted a house where they could stay and have supervised feeding. I set the student midwives to work growing vegetables and caring for chickens, so we could offer them some decent food. Meanwhile, Sister Belinda gave their mothers basic lessons in cooking nutritious meals. A great favourite was her rice pudding. Rice was part of the staple Malawian diet, but they never put milk in it. The mothers watched in great amazement as Sister Belinda added milk and sugar to iron-fortified rice, thereby transforming a pretty nutrition-free meal for growing children. As far as I know, milky rice pudding has gone down in the region's history!

As our first Christmas approached we wanted to give the student midwives a small gift, but we were rather stuck on what to choose. We didn't know how they would receive a present, whether they would then feel obliged to give us something back in return, or what the custom was. It seemed quite a delicate issue, but we really did want to give them just a little something each. As we sat at the dinner table one night, Sister Belinda had a brainwave.

'I know, why don't we give them an umbrella each?'

'Oh yes, well, there's an idea,' Sister Marie-Louise said.

The students hated getting their beloved uniforms wet in the tropical downpours as they rushed from their house to the hospital. I loved the way they took such great care of them, keeping them totally spotless (which was difficult because Malawi was so dusty) and pressed (unlike some of their British counterparts!). So we ordered 20 big, sturdy umbrellas, in a range of the brightest primary colours. On Christmas Eve we wrapped each one and labelled them, and left them on the beds of each of the student midwives.

That night as the time approached for Midnight Mass, we could hear a rising sound of singing coming from all directions. We looked out of the window and could see tiny pinpricks of swinging lights in the dark night as the people came down from their villages to church, all singing their own carols. It was a beautiful start to Christmas, to be surrounded by such uninhibited, joyful devotion; it was, I think, the most meaningful Midnight Mass I have ever experienced.

By breakfast time on Christmas Day, however, we still had heard nothing about our umbrellas.

'Gosh, I hope they haven't taken offence!' Sister Belinda said.

'I hope they know what they are,' I added.

'Oh, look!' Sister Marie-Louise exclaimed, pointing out of the window.

The students were coming out of their accommodation in a long line, each holding their umbrella and singing as they came up the path. We followed behind them, intrigued and a little anxious as to what they were going to do next.

They walked into the main quad up to the big tree where we had a crib displayed and made a circle around it. The little student at the front stepped forward to face the crib, bowed and showed her big green umbrella. Then her face broke into a grin and she said, 'Look, Jesus! Look at my umbrella. It is good. Thank you, Jesus!'

Then she put it back down and walked back to the circle, and the next student stepped forward and did the same with her big red umbrella, 'Jesus, this is my umbrella. See how it works. Thank you, Jesus, thank you for my beautiful umbrella!'

And so it went on until every one of the 20 students had presented their umbrellas to baby Jesus. The umbrellas went on to be treasured by their new owners.

Gradually the items on the list I had written on my first night were getting crossed off – I had set up the midwifery training school, the Land Rover was increasingly used as a mobile clinic to give antenatal and post-natal services to the remote villages, the hospital facilities were gradually being upgraded (we had addressed the 'failure to walk' problem by clearing one of the outbuildings and opening it to heavily pregnant women to come and live in simply, in the one or two weeks before their babies were due), and plans were well underway to build a proper operating theatre.

Because there was no such thing as a national health service in Malawi, everyone had to pay to use the hospital. Obviously, most people didn't have any money. To help, we introduced a scheme where every time they came to the antenatal clinic, the money they paid for their visit was offset against the actual delivery. This meant there was a great incentive for mothers to come in for their checks and we avoided quite a few medical problems later, and most people did not have to pay for the birth of their babies.

But one thing that I felt was still desperately needed was a special baby-care unit for the babies who needed intensive care because they were either born very prematurely or were acutely vulnerable. Our resources were very limited. In the hospitals I'd worked in, back in England, the neonatal units had proper incubators, monitors and breathing and resuscitation equipment. Here, all we could manage was a higher staff-to-baby ratio, hot-water bottles for the night, a fan for the day and specially made tiny clothes. Really, it was about keeping a closer eye on them, their feeding and weight, and guarding them more carefully against infection. However, we felt that this was better than nothing and lives would still be saved, so we got the room set up. We had room for ten babies and it seemed to be helping.

But in newborn babies, particularly those who have been born prematurely, the greatest threat they face is infection. Of course in Malawi we were surrounded by so many more dangerous diseases than at home. I didn't really know how we could protect these vulnerable babies except by strictly limiting those who could come into the room to the mothers only, and forbidding anyone who had the slightest cough, sneeze, sore throat or – the biggest threat in Malawi, diarrhoea and vomiting – to come in. So I always had someone on the door with a checklist of questions.

'Which baby are you coming to see?'

'What relation are you to the baby?'

'In the last 24 hours, have you had a sore throat?'

'Have you had a cough?'

'Have you got catarrh?'

'Have you had a temperature?'

'Have you had diarrhoea or vomiting?'

And lastly, 'Have you washed your hands?'

These questions were a constant hum in the background of the special-care unit like a kind of backing track, and I always had an ear open for them, to make sure they were being asked. One day, I was in there and I was vaguely aware of the reassuring sound of the usual checks taking place, when suddenly one of the mothers shouted, 'She was sick this morning. She lied! I saw her.'

She was pointing at one of the other mothers, who was stroking her baby lying in her cot. My heart sank.

I went over.

'Is this true?'

She nodded.

'You have put your baby in grave danger. You must leave straight away,' I said.

She left the unit but it was too late. Within a short time her baby started to get sick and within 48 hours, she was dead. One by one, all the babies started to get ill. We worked so hard. All the nurses and Sister Marie-Louise came in to help, but it was no good. Within a few days many of the babies were dead.

Soon the hospital was filled with the most terrible wailing. The Malawian people had their ways of expressing grief, which were loud and dramatic. Sister Marie-Louise and I were quiet, in a state of shock. We didn't know what to do or where to put ourselves. The staff didn't know what to do with us either. In the end they took our hands and led us out to the big tree in the centre of the quad, where we usually met for prayer. They sat us down and stood facing us, and started to quietly sing hymns for us. They sang until the sun went down and the moon rose. Thoughts of my father and his resilience came into my head. In the end I stood up and said a prayer for the women who had lost their babies, and then said:

Bless us God, Keep us safe in your encircling arms, with the bright moon that is above us, and the warm earth beneath our feet. Hold us and protect us through the friends who surround us and in our knowledge of you living in our hearts. Amen.

And I went into the house and went to bed, exhausted, in the hope of a better day.

Going to Malawi was the most amazing experience. I grew and I changed; I found an energy and resourcefulness that I didn't know I had. But it came at a price. By the start of my fourth year I was exhausted and sleep-deprived. The work was relentless; we could only handle a fraction of the mothers who came to us. The sheer scale of the help that was needed was frightening and I began to become overwhelmed with the feeling that whatever we did, we could only scratch the surface. The money, resources and manpower were not there. And most of all, I began to get ill. I had suffered from diarrhoea from the moment I arrived, but I got sicker and sicker, my guts were rotting. I felt I could not stay much longer in Malawi, but I also could not imagine myself back in England, or even back in the Community after being so free. So at the beginning of my fourth year I wrote to Mother Sarah Grace:

> *Dear Mother,*
>
> *I am writing to tell you I can no longer continue with my work at St Anne's Hospital. I am exhausted and I am ill. I am also concerned that I am going to find it very difficult to return to life in the Community after four years away, and I am not sure how to go on living the religious life.*

A week later, we received a wire saying that Mother Sarah Grace was on her way over to see us. I felt terribly guilty: it wasn't a short trip. But when she arrived, a few weeks later, it was not with the reaction I expected. I think she did not know what to say to me or how to handle the situation; I felt as if I had become a stranger to her. For a start she didn't seem to want to speak to me. Mother Sarah Grace spent most of her time in St John's

House with Sister Belinda. Of course I was terribly busy in the hospital so unless she came down to find me, our paths wouldn't cross. When I finally did have a meeting with her, it seemed terribly formal. I longed to hear some loving concern and care in her voice. Instead she sat opposite me impassively as I explained that I was exhausted and ill.

'Well, you have just got to get on with it,' she said.

'I don't think I can carry on, Mother.'

'In which case you will have to come home.'

'But I'm not sure I want or even can come home now. As I said in my letter to you, I don't know how I can return to Community life or perhaps even stay in the religious life. Being here has changed me absolutely.'

'Sister Catherine Mary, you made formal vows to God. You cannot seriously consider breaking them. No, I can see, you need to come home straight away.'

And that was it. Before I knew it, I was packing my bags and Sister Sarah Jane was on her way out from England to replace me. It was heartbreaking. Anton was in tears: 'Goodbye, Mama,' he said, bowing and then he broke my heart by bursting into the first verse of one of my favourite hymns,

Abide with me, fast falls the eventide;
the darkness deepens; Lord, with me abide:
when other helpers fail, and comforts flee,
help of the helpless, O abide with me.

I'm not sure what I had been looking for from Mother Sarah Grace. Maybe some understanding, some recognition of what I had been through, that I had tried my hardest and yes, maybe some praise. I think I definitely needed to feel someone cared, that I was cherished in some way and concern could be felt for me. Sometimes I had felt these things from our Reverend Mother and indeed the rest of the Community, but on this occasion I didn't. I was left feeling like I had failed.

A year later, when we had completed our five years, the Sisters packed up, handed over the hospital to the diocese and national midwives, and came home.

CHAPTER ELEVEN

WORKING IN A MYSTERIOUS WAY

I sat in the quiet ward and looked at the clock. I decided to say a prayer.

> *Dear God, If I am supposed to take a job at the British Hospital, send the midwife tutor to come and find me. If she doesn't appear, I will know this is not the path you want me to take. Amen.*

That felt about right, but I couldn't help glancing at the clock every so often, trying to second-guess when she might finish her talk and appear. I was supposed to go and listen to the senior midwifery tutor from the British Hospital for Mothers and Babies. She had come to give a talk to the midwives at the Lambeth Hospital, where I had a temporary job. But that evening I found myself on the rota to be on call with the 'bleep'. I was a bit ambivalent about this; I had finished my reorientation to British obstetrics and I was looking for a job as a tutor. I knew that the British Hospital had a position going.

It was a hospital with a Christian foundation, so in theory it should have been perfect for me. But it was known to be on the evangelical wing of the Church and I was concerned that as a Sister in a religious Community (and therefore likely seen to be more Anglo-Catholic), I might not fit in so I hadn't made any enquiries.

Now, sitting in the dark ward, I honestly didn't know whether I wanted her to appear or not, but I did want an answer either way. Anyway, every time someone went past the door I jumped. Eventually the time came for the end of my shift. 'Too late now,' I thought to myself. 'Oh well, that's that then.' So I went off to the nurses' kitchen, made myself a cup of tea, kicked off my shoes and curled up on the sofa in the sitting room. I felt neither happy nor sad, just like something had been decided. Then the senior midwifery tutor from the British Hospital walked in.

'Sister Catherine Mary?'

'Yes,' I replied.

'Hello. I'm Anne, the head of midwifery at the British Hospital.'

'Yes', I stuttered.

'I believe you may be looking for a tutor's post?'

'Yes'. I was so astonished that I was literally rendered mute but she didn't seem to notice, or at least it didn't put her off. She went on to invite me to come and look round the next week. The next thing I knew I'd been for an interview and been offered a job as obstetric nurse tutor. This turned out to be the best thing that ever happened to me.

When I got back to England from Malawi at the end of 1974, I was in a bad way. Because Mother Sarah Grace had told me I couldn't do so, I had put any idea of renouncing my vows out of my mind. I did, however, need rest and had to go through extensive medical investigations for my illness. With expert treatment I gradually got better and began to regain a sense of purpose.

While I recovered, I returned to work at the Lambeth Hospital and because things had moved on a bit in the world of midwifery while I was abroad, I concentrated on updating my midwifery skills. I had spent four intense years working in such a different environment, having to think on my feet, doing things such as tying up pelvises with luggage straps and performing impromptu proce-dures that would not have been allowed here, that I felt I had to be reorientated (or perhaps reconditioned) to the British system.

I was struck by how much more medicalised birth had become in the four years I'd been away. Of course it's on a whole different scale now, but even back in 1974 the world was becoming more litigious. I noticed that midwives were referring up to the doctors' decisions that ten years before they would have taken responsibility for themselves. This meant doctors were a greater presence in the delivery room. But I'd changed as well. I noticed I was much more confident; I was far more certain in my analysis of what was going on in labour and delivery. I felt I was a much better midwife.

In 1978 I began work as the obstetrics tutor at the British Hospital. I was on the bottom rung of the teaching ladder, but from the moment I started, I loved it. The hospital was in Woolwich and the people, while not East Enders in the 'born within the sound of Bow Bells' sense, had every attribute of the true East Ender – the warmth, gregariousness, humour (let's call it earthy) and, of course, the fondness for a flutter. They were the East Enders South of the River, really. Some of the buildings had changed, though. I couldn't get over the Thamesmead Estate. Long ago, when I was training as a midwife, I had learned to drive, hurtling around doing figures of eight with my instructor shouting at me from the passenger seat, on the derelict land that ran alongside the Thames at Woolwich. When I returned, this land had been turned into the huge Thamesmead Estate. Miles of concrete blocks raised off the marshy ground on columns, connected by high-level walkways, designed to house 60,000 to 100,000 people. It was cut off by large roads, and what should have been a model new modern estate seemed to incubate a whole range of social problems.

The rest of Woolwich was, by contrast, rather suburban and friendly. The hospital itself was very elegant and welcoming. I loved the way it had a beautiful drive surrounded by immaculately kept gardens and the fact that the chapel was straight in front of you when you entered, right at the very heart. It was all very small, contained and friendly, with a common purpose. We could get out into the gardens easily and when the weather was good, we used to throw open the doors and sit and have our lessons outside underneath a big tree surrounded by flowers.

I think this common purpose of striving to have God at the centre of our lives and expressing this in our vocation caring for the local people meant we existed happily, with a very good working relationship, with the doctors. My worries about my different religious approach were unfounded, I immediately felt accepted and loved. I became lifelong friends with some of the tutors there, two of whom I still go on holiday with every year, and the small size of the hospital meant I got to know my students well. Because the British Hospital had a Christian foundation, many of the students had either been missionaries or were training to go out and be midwives in the developing world. So I often set aside ten minutes at the end of my lectures to talk about how what we had learned that day could be applied abroad. It felt good to be able to pass on the knowledge I had gained in Malawi.

I think the Christian ethos brought something special to the patients too. We used to ask the new parents if they would like to have a little thanksgiving service for themselves and their babies. Most mothers were delighted, even if they weren't Christian.

It was just a little service in the chapel if the mother could manage it, or beside her bed if she couldn't, and it replaced the old service of 'churching', which can still be found in the Book of Common Prayer. Childbirth used to be such a risky business for both mother and baby that a special blessing would be said over the mother 40 days after she had given birth. The traditional service has elements of ritual purification and echoes of the ancient rule that a woman could not go back to church until she had been 'churched'. In the old days a mother would often come into the church wearing a veil and carrying a candle, and would sit on a special 'churching' seat at the back. She would be expected to make an offering and then the priest would bless her as she knelt at the altar.

Our service was much more straightforward – a couple of readings, a special prayer and a special blessing. I think we dismiss our ancient rituals too readily. Bringing new life to the world is still the most extraordinary event in a woman's life, probably *the* most important event, and to mark it in some way, some official way, with thanksgiving, where those closest to her can participate, is precious. Our service of thanksgiving always seemed to be much appreciated.

Another much-loved part of the life at the British Hospital was our annual nativity tableau. Eight evenings before Christmas, the hospital staff would tell the

Christmas story through Bible readings, acting and singing. We tended to use the same script – as one of the more 'mature' ladies on the staff, I always played Elizabeth, the mother of John the Baptist. Students and midwives played Mary, Joseph and the shepherds and kings, and the baby Jesus would be one of our babies that had just been born. It was a great honour for your new baby to be asked to play Jesus, and I don't remember any mother ever refusing!

So the British Hospital was a special place where I felt at home and I have to say these were the happiest days of my life. After a few years I had worked my way up through various tutoring posts and eventually I became the senior midwifery tutor. I had arrived back from Malawi with no idea what to do next, but I felt as if my patience and faith in God had been rewarded. In the words of the famous hymn, 'God works in a mysterious way His wonders to perform'.

However, the winds of change were continuing to blow and the National Health Service was evolving at a pace. As the Eighties progressed, the government was pursuing a policy (which of course it still is) where the various small, often specialist, hospitals which had sprung up piecemeal over the years were gradually closing and merged with larger, more general, hospitals. Of course there were advantages to this. Just as an example, at the British Hospital we had a special-care baby unit, but there was a limit to the amount of equipment we had at our disposal and we didn't have the money to be able to give our babies some of the more complicated treatments or expertise they could get at a bigger hospital and sometimes they had to be transferred. So it wasn't a surprise when there was an announcement that the British Hospital was to be merged with the Greenwich District Hospital. In practice this meant that the hospital had to close and we would all have to move to Greenwich. We were devastated. While we knew there were obvious advantages to the merger, our community and ethos would be diluted in the huge pool of a secular general hospital. Also, we had the impression that the feelings were mutual. Some of the staff at the district hospital were not really looking forward to having us either.

This feeling was shared by some of our patients. Mrs Miller had had her two sons at the British (one of whom I had been in charge of) and visiting one day, she mentioned that she and her husband were thinking of trying for another baby in the New Year.

'Well, you'll have to get a move on if you want it here,' I said, 'This hospital will be closed by July.'

Mrs Miller obviously went home and rethought her timing with Mr Miller because almost exactly nine months later, and a week before the hospital closed, I delivered Mary Miller.

So with great regret in the summer of 1984 we had our big final service in the chapel and I found myself working on the maternity wards of Greenwich District

Hospital. But the British was not forgotten. One day, as I was looking at a noticeboard, I felt a tap on my shoulder.

'Excuse me, Sister Catherine Mary, isn't it?'

'Yes, dear.'

'Do you remember me?'

I gave her a thorough inspection.

'Well, I think I do recognise you. Did you have a baby at the British Hospital?'

'Yes, that's me. I'm Clare.'

'Hello, Clare, how can I help you?'

'Well, I'm a bit embarrassed to ask.'

'Don't worry. Go ahead!'

'Well, you didn't deliver my baby but you did a service of thanksgiving for him, and it was really good. I wondered whether you could do the same again for my new baby girl? Doesn't seem right him having it and not her. Only I asked and they said they don't do it here.'

'Well, no, they don't. Not normally. But I don't see why we can't have one anyway. Leave it with me.'

So I went and talked to the hospital chaplain and later on that afternoon, we did a special thanksgiving for Clare and her new baby. It was a happy moment, but also a sad reminder of what we had lost at the British Hospital.

However, there was something, or rather someone, that I found as a result of the move to Greenwich. I was waiting at the reception desk when I became aware of a nurse standing next to me. I turned and looked, and I nearly passed out. Beside me was a ghost. I was looking at the profile of Cecilia. She didn't notice me, but as I stared, I was sure I was looking at a slightly aged (but not that much) Cecilia, dressed not in a habit, but in the uniform of a district nurse. As I paused, the thought crossed my mind that I could just slip away. I touched her arm instead.

'Cecilia!'

She turned and the colour drained from her face.

'Catherine!'

And then I found myself all overcome and hugging her.

'Oh, I never thought I'd see you again! It's so good to see you!'

'It's so good to see you too, Catherine. I think of you every day and wonder how you are. And here you are.'

She drew back and looked at me, and then looked at my girdle and habit.

'So you've taken final vows?'

'Yes – some years ago.'

'I'm so glad.'

'*Are* you?'

Suddenly the conversation seemed to be getting into dangerous territory; it hadn't taken long. How quickly that unresolved bit of anger about her departure could rise to the surface, as fresh and dangerous as the day she'd left! I needed to ask her some questions.

'Cecilia, can we go and talk? There's lots of things I want to know.'

She looked concerned, but she said, 'Yes, I think that would be good.'

There were all sorts of things I was supposed to be doing, but I thought this was one occasion where God would forgive me putting my own needs first. In fact, as we walked to the hospital canteen, I wondered what God's purpose might be for Cecilia and I to meet again now.

We sat down with an ordinary cup of tea and piece of cake and started to have an extraordinary conversation. I had to get the big one out of the way straight away, almost just in case she disappeared again.

'Why did you leave?' I asked.

She took a breath and sighed.

'Because I couldn't carry on any longer. I didn't want to be a midwife. As you know, I'd never wanted to be a midwife, but I felt that I had to give it a go. I prayed and prayed, but the answer came back the same. My calling was to be a district nurse.'

'But it was so sudden. Why didn't you talk to me?'

'Perhaps I should have done, but I suppose I didn't want to interfere with what definitely was your calling … and I was in shock.'

'*Shock*?'

Cecilia then told me how she had been sent to deliver a baby at short notice. When she went into the room her instincts were telling her that something was seriously wrong. In the event there was something terribly wrong – the baby was lying in a breech position and had died. She had never seen a stillborn baby before and no one had prepared her for what to expect.

'I handled it really badly, but the last straw was when I bumped into Sister Julia in the corridor afterwards and she said, "I hear you had a breech birth today. That was good experience for you." I felt she hadn't understood the emotional impact this had had on me and the poor mother.'

I nodded. I could picture the scene only too well. Cecilia then told me how she had gone back to the Mission House and been unable to do anything but go to meals for two days. Her predicament wasn't helped by overhearing Sister Alice talking about a lady in the parish whom she'd had to make a post-natal visit to, despite the fact that her baby was stillborn, and this lady had told her how the inexperienced midwife did not know what she was doing and had panicked.

'That was me,' Cecilia said. 'It confirmed what I had always believed – I did not want to be a midwife and my calling was to be a district nurse, something the Community was not prepared at that time to let me do.'

We sat in silence for a few minutes. I felt the enormity of what Cecilia had just told me. Then she continued.

'I searched my soul but I felt my time in Community had come to an end and I had to leave. In the end, it really wasn't a choice.'

'No, I can see that. You know I needed to hear you tell me this.'

Cecilia looked at me intently for a second and then said, 'I have never regretted leaving the religious life but

I have regretted the way I left, and particularly the way I never had the chance to explain or say goodbye to you and the Sisters.'

'Well, I guess God has given us the chance to make up for that now,' I said and we embraced.

I never saw Cecilia again, but we started to write to each other and we are still in contact. It really did make a difference, meeting her again. I no longer felt angry towards her – how could I after hearing her story? But meeting her only added to my feelings of discomfort with the some aspects of our Community life, not just the fact we were not allowed to say 'goodbye' properly and the thinking that lay behind it, but also the weight that was given (or not given) to our own feelings about where God was calling us. But for the moment I kept those thoughts to myself.

CHAPTER TWELVE
REVOLUTION

Sometimes I did worry about the future. I could see that there was a fundamental crisis looming for the religious life. The world that had given birth to monks and nuns was rapidly becoming history. The most obvious symptom of this crisis was the fall not just in numbers of people going to church, but also entering and remaining in the religious life, and our Community was no exception. No new Sisters had joined since Sister Marie-Louise.

But this fall in numbers was mirrored by an identity crisis. Many felt that to cling onto a lifestyle created in the last century seemed inappropriate. But what should take its place? Each Community had its own way of engaging with the changing world and we were no exception. Although I continued working as a midwife tutor in hospital and living in a Community House in London, things began to move within the Community itself.

Mother Sarah Grace could be quite secretive sometimes. One day in 1976 she announced she was off on a day trip.

'Where's she off to?' the Sisters asked each other, but no one seemed to know the answer.

When the Reverend Mother got back late in the evening, she summoned Sister Rachel and Sister Julia into her study and waved a piece of paper at them.

'A week ago I received this letter and it's been burning a hole in my pocket. It's from Mother Theresa Mary in Birmingham. Their House there is now far too big for them and they want to rejoin their Mother House in Oxfordshire. Mother Theresa Mary was wondering whether we might be interested in taking it over.'

'Oh Mother, not Birmingham!' Poor Sister Rachel exclaimed before she could stop herself.

'Well yes, indeed Birmingham. However, I've been up there today and I think it might suit our purposes perfectly.'

'Really?'

'Yes. And that's why I want both of you to go up and see it with me soon.'

Sisters Rachel and Julia exchanged pained glances but to no avail. A week later they had to pile into the Community car with the Reverend Mother, muttering darkly to each other about how they could have understood London, but Birmingham? None of us came from the Midlands and the Community had never worked there. We had absolutely no connection whatsoever with the city, and no particular desire to form one.

However, as soon as the Sisters had got out of the car and gone over the threshold of the Birmingham House, they knew they had found our new Mother House. It was a large eighteenth-century farmhouse, complete with a garden and a chapel, set in a deprived area of the inner city. This would be an oasis of peace, in the middle of a busy, needy community, with lots of things for us to do. It was a cunning move by the Reverend Mother to take Sister Rachel and Sister Julia with her because they were respected representatives of both the modernising and conservative factions within the Community; with the support of them both, she knew she would carry the other Sisters. Within the year we had said goodbye to our Mother House in Hastings and moved from the quiet, enchanted forest to an urban jungle in the middle of Birmingham.

This move wasn't a total shock. Every five years religious Communities receive a 'visitation' from their Bishop. This is a kind of audit of the Community's life and work, where every member of the Community is interviewed about what they do, and their thoughts about the Community's future. In 1975 the Bishop of Chichester spent some time looking at the Mother House and at the end of it, he took Mother Sarah Grace aside.

'Look, I'm the last person who wants to see you leave my Diocese,' he said, 'but you need to get into the thick of it. This nursing home is taking up all your energy and has a stranglehold on your future. You need to find a new home and a new purpose.'

And the Bishop was right: we were facing a crossroads in the life of the Community. To understand the depth of it, you have to go back to the years immediately following the Second World War. Two pivotal things happened. In 1945 the Sisters were finally allowed to take life vows. Up until this time they had not been allowed to enter the religious life in the fullest, most permanent sense, although they had been living it.

Because the Community of St John the Divine had been set up primarily as a nursing Community, and an Anglican one at that, the religious element had originally only been a means to a more professional nursing end. In fact, because of the anti-Catholic feeling in the British establishment, any attempts by the Sisters to become more formally religious had been strenuously resisted. It was felt that this would both deter women from entering the Community and end in popery.

In reality, most of the women who had joined the Community were deeply religious and longed to be able to express this more formally. They were living the life of the fully professed and wanted to make a public commitment to God. Finally, with great rejoicing among the Sisters, they managed to persuade the church authorities to let them take their life vows. On 2 October 1945, the Feast of the Holy Guardian Angels, most of the Sisters took their life vows. Three Sisters did not, but all of them stayed living in the Community for the rest of their lives, abiding by the three vows, even though they hadn't publicly professed them.

Meanwhile, in 1947 the National Health Service Act was passed and came into effect in 1948. However, it took a long time for the big, overarching beast that we now know as the NHS to emerge. Rather than a revolution and takeover, it was more like a slow expansion and creeping colonisation of the services that were already there. This meant that our work as nurses and midwives carried on as it had done for many years, with the funding that previously came direct from our patients or charitable donations gradually being taken over by the NHS. Then in 1974 the Sisters started to become individual employees of the Health Service. Looking back now, it was obvious that the writing was on the wall.

Well, Mother Sarah Grace didn't shirk from this new challenge: she knew the Bishop was right. Although we were doing good work in the nursing home and would have quite happily carried on, the rising cost of staff and supplies meant that we could only look after the relatively comfortably off, rather than the people who really needed us. After much discussion and prayer it was decided that the Mother House should be sold and we should look for somewhere that we could start a new ministry. We had no idea what this ministry should be except that perhaps it could still involve health and healing, but in a wider, more holistic sense.

And it was not only our Mother House in Hastings that had to close. Our work in London seemed to be coming to an end. In 1978 our lease on the Mission House was up for renewal. It had originally been given to us for a token rent by the Diocese in 1945 after our Bow Lane house was destroyed by the bomb that killed Sister Margery. Now the Church wanted a more economically realistic rent, which we had no means of paying. As the NHS expanded its midwifery training, the numbers of pupil midwives coming to train with us dwindled and we had no option but to close down the Mission House.

It was a sad time. The local community were dismayed – we had been present at births, cared for the sick and laid out their dead for 100 years. A petition was sent to the Bishop from the people of Poplar, but we had to accept that we were no longer needed. Our prayers had been answered and now our work there was complete. So we packed up the Mission House (no easy job, it took months), sent lots of our stuff to the City Mission for the Homeless, and became nomads in the London desert. We stayed for a little while in a small vicarage in Bow that smelt of cats, and then shared a house in Vauxhall.

Some Sisters became part of a mixed religious Community in Limehouse. The Community was no longer directly employed by the NHS and the houses we lived in were no longer clinics, but rather centres of prayer to which we returned each evening after work. It meant that Sisters who worked in hospitals had the use of cars, which was exciting! But it was a very different kind of communal living to when we had all been working together as a team in the Mission House. Sometimes I felt we were a bit like the Israelites, wandering round the desert during the exodus from Egypt, looking for a permanent home.

So there was a sense of a pending crisis. But when I use the word 'crisis' I don't necessarily mean this in a negative way. The Chinese written word for 'crisis' is made up of two characters – one is 'danger' and the other is 'opportunity' – and I really see this as having been a tricky, scary and yet exciting time for the Sisters.

For many years the move to Birmingham had little impact on me. I stayed in London, commuting from whichever temporary residence we were living in to my work as a midwife tutor. I loved it and I felt as if I was finally truly fulfilling my vocation. But then the winds of change hit me personally. The government changed the laws regarding nursing and midwifery training. Before, training to become a midwife had been a certificated course with a weekly study day and planned working on the different ward areas the rest of the week. It meant we got to know the students and witnessed how they worked, while maintaining our own competency by working. Perhaps most importantly, it gave the students a very good grounding in the basics. But at the end of the 1980s legislation was passed that removed training from the hospitals and required every midwife to go to college or university.

This, in fact, has much to commend it and I have nothing against student midwives going to university. But not everyone can be a high-flyer. Some women are more practically minded, some are not academic or they have other commitments like families of their own, but this doesn't mean that they wouldn't make excellent midwives. Yes, you have to have the basic medical and obstetric knowledge, but being a midwife is so much more than that – it's about intuition, experience and the ability to connect with a mother – things that university can't teach, that are actually best taught out on the ward. It also meant that whereas there used to be a good number of student midwives on the wards now, apart from their placements some of their work would have to be undertaken by much less trained healthcare assistants. I would also have to go back and study for further academic qualifications. This would have been difficult while teaching full time and living the religious life and, quite frankly, after years of teaching and working in obstetrics, I didn't want to do it.

After much prayer and heart searching, disillusioned and generally at a low ebb, I handed in my notice and asked for some time to pray. While doing this, I needed something practical to do so I put on some rubber gloves and an apron and started cleaning the house in Vauxhall. I thought I'd get through a couple of rooms before some sort of inspiration struck. In the end I was at it for a year and managed to scrub the whole house from top to bottom. I started at the top and worked my way through every room – washing down walls, scrubbing floors, polishing doorknobs, praying all the time. In the end the Vauxhall house was immaculate, but my soul remained pretty murky. I felt as if I was bereaved and I kept weeping into my bucket. I couldn't believe God really wanted me to give up midwifery, but whichever way round I looked at it, that was the message I was getting.

I was finally put out of my misery when the Holy Spirit arrived in the form of a book, *Holy Listening: The Art of Spiritual Direction* by Margaret Guenther. I read it straight through, starting in the morning and going right through the day into the night, until I had read it four times without stopping. The answer to my predicament was written right there, loud and clear. At the beginning of the book there was a quote from the medieval mystic Eckhart, and this is what caught my attention:

> *Tend only to the birth in you and you will find all goodness and all consolation, all delight, all being and all truth. Reject it and you reject goodness and blessing. What comes to you in this birth brings with it pure being and blessing. But what you seek or love outside of this birth will come to nothing, no matter what you will or where you will it.*

The book spoke to me about how I might become a different kind of midwife, to help give birth to something perhaps more profound and eternal. As Margaret Guenther said in her book:

The birth of God in the soul is our own true birth and the midwife is the person who is with the birthgiver, standing alongside at a time of vulnerability, deep and intimate, the guardian of new life, keeping safe, helping bring to birth. She does things with, not to, the birthgiver, she teaches in the best sense of the word, in that she helps the birthgiver towards ever greater self-knowledge.

I really felt that this was what the Holy Spirit was calling me to, being a midwife of the soul. I started praying about becoming a spiritual director. Perhaps the best way to describe this is as someone who walks alongside others as they attempt to deepen their relationship with God. So I made some enquiries and started my training.

And that was what I thought I was meant to do. However, I should have known by now that God likes to throw in surprises.

At the end of that year, 1991, Mother Sarah Grace announced that she was coming to the end of her term of office and would not be standing for re-election as Reverend Mother. This was no surprise; by now she was in her seventies and had been looking after us all for a very long time. It meant there was to be an election chapter. There were no nominations – the name of every Sister who had been life professed for more than six years and was under the age of 70 automatically went on to the ballot paper. The whole process was overseen by the Chaplain General and, in accordance with tradition, Mother Sarah Grace was not present at the election chapter, but gave her vote privately to the Chaplain beforehand.

On the big day, in ominous silence, we all filed into the Chapel. It was the first election of a Superior I had ever taken part in and there was a feeling of solemnity surrounding the whole occasion. No one was making eye contact. 'Hmm, a good day for custody of the eyes,' I thought to myself. But I was pretty sure I could predict how most of them would be voting.

It seemed a very big deal to vote for a new Mother. Mother Sarah Grace, whom from today would be known simply as Sister Sarah Grace, had been such a towering figure in the Community for so long. She really had been a mother to all of us. I couldn't imagine who could take her place and have the same authority. It was actually quite scary – like having a rug pulled from under your feet. The new Mother would guide the direction of the Community for years to come, and I was under no illusion how difficult the choices were for whoever took over.

As I've said, the whole Community was in the middle of a prolonged time of discernment and change. Like any arena where decisions have to be made, there were sides – there were the conservatives and then there were the modernisers. Of course I was on the modernising wing of the Community and I was going to vote for my old mentor, Sister Rachel, as a humane and forward-thinking choice. My catastrophic fantasy was that Sister Julia would get the job and that would put me in a difficult position as regards my future with the Community. But looking at the circle of Sisters around me I thought that on balance the wish for change outweighed the wish to maintain the status quo, and my catastrophic fantasy would remain a fantasy.

The Chaplain said a prayer and then we went up, one by one, and handed him our votes.

We remained in the chapel waiting, all of us kneeling in silent prayer, as the Chaplain retired to a separate room to count the votes. After 15 minutes or so, which seemed an eternity, he came in and standing in front of us, as we stayed with our heads bowed, said a prayer and then announced, 'Having counted the votes, I am pleased to announce that the new Reverend Mother of this Community of St John the Divine is Sister Catherine Mary. May God bless you, Mother Catherine Mary!'

I felt myself sway on my knees. Did I just hear that right? I must have done, because everyone was turning and looking at me and smiling. Community folklore had it that when Mother Sarah Grace was elected, she remained on her knees praying in silence in the chapel for hours.

I jumped up and strode out of the chapel back to my room, in a state of shock and tearful.

The Chaplain General came in and seeing I obviously wasn't too happy, said, 'Can I make you a cup of tea?'

'I think I need something stronger than that,' I replied.

Then the former Mother Sarah Grace paid a visit.

'You are surprised?'

'Surprised? I'll say! I never thought it would be me. I've never even held an Office in the Community. What on earth's going on?'

'It was obvious to me.'

'Obvious to *you*? You didn't say. You could have warned me.'

She looked at me quizzically.

'I can go on sabbatical if it would make things easier for you,' she said.

I was shocked.

'No, there's no need for that. I don't think I shall be inhibited by your presence.'

'No, you never have been and that is why you are the right person for the job. You will be in my prayers.' And with that she left.

I slipped out and rang my mother to tell her.

'Well, *you* asked for it,' she said.

'That's the whole point, Mother. I didn't.'

'Hmm. Well, I hope you haven't bitten off more than you can chew.'

'Mother, are you listening? It was bitten off for me!'

I gave up and hung up. Mothers can be so frustrating.

The last person to visit was Sister Rachel.

'I never wanted this. I'm not a leader, I'm just a junior member of this Community,' I said.

'That's why we voted for you. We need someone younger, with the vision and courage to take us to places we never dreamt of. It's the only way we are going to grow. Jesus's way wasn't easy and he caused absolute havoc, but look what he achieved.'

'You are not reassuring me, Rachel! He ended up on the Cross.'

'And saving us all.'

For the first time since the election I managed to smile.

'I didn't want this. I thought I was going to be a spiritual director.'

'And you can still be a spiritual director. But you also have the opportunity to help give birth to a whole new Community. Think about it; it's so exciting. And I will be with you every step of the way.'

She took my hand.

'How on earth am I going to do this?' I asked her.

'One step at a time,' she said and went to the door. She then added, 'What doesn't kill you makes you stronger.'

'I never knew what part of the Bible that's from.'

'It isn't. It's Nietzsche,' she said and left smiling.

The next morning I went downstairs into the Reverend Mother's office and tried sitting behind her desk. Suddenly I felt a lot more brave and purposeful. I thought very hard about all the things that I felt should define us, and all the things that were superfluous and got in the way of our ministry in the modern world, and then I wrote a list. At the top of it was the word 'Habits'.

I knew this might be just tinkering at the edges, but it seemed a relatively safe place to start!

To be fair, things had been moving in the right direction for a while. It all started with a rather disastrous camping holiday in the Lake District. Sisters Alice and Sarah Jane had climbed up Helvellyn in a gale in their habits and had nearly taken off. At the next chapter meeting they put forward a motion that in future they should be allowed to wear ordinary sensible clothes on holiday. It was overwhelmingly passed and after that there was a flood of exceptions put forward at every chapter meeting – for example, that the parentcraft classes should be done in trousers (it was most unseemly to be messing around on the floor and bending over people in a skirt). By the time I became the Reverend Mother, we were allowed to wear normal clothes on our days off, but we still had to get changed for chapel.

The first thing I did was order wardrobes to be fitted in each of the bedrooms. Our new 'mufti' required previously unneeded hanging space. Marie-Louise, Rachel and I were currently sharing a cupboard in the corridor. And as no one seemed to mind this very much, I then raised the issue in chapter of making the wearing of habits optional at all times. What mattered was what was inside, our vows and commitment and the way we lived our lives; our cross and our ring symbolised the consecration we had made. Perhaps we would have to work harder if we couldn't hide behind a habit. It was also sometimes a barrier, marking us out. The motion was passed with a solid majority. I was surprised how readily the Sisters agreed to come out of the habit. Only two remained in them – Sister Belinda and Sister Julia, and that was fine. It was only optional.

Then in the same spirit I suggested that we stopped having to address each other as Sister and I definitely did not want to be called Mother. That was more difficult to get through, but I kept arguing these words can be barriers to each other. We are human beings like every one else: even if we have formally put Christ at the very centre of our existence, we need to take away everything that separates us from each other and the wider community. It was passed with a slender majority.

From the very beginning I had been concerned that some things in our way of life could impede the Sisters from growing in maturity. I wanted us to take more responsibility for the direction of our ministries and that meant giving everyone more freedom to think and choose. We collectively decided to give everyone a budget of £30 a month for personal use. In some ways it was just a token amount, but it made a huge difference. I noticed the value of things for a start and it was a relief not to have to request our personal toiletries on a list. But the best thing was being able to buy small gifts – a chocolate bar for a birthday, a book to say thank you.

Along with rights come responsibilities. We changed the decision-making process so that we became much more democratic with far more decisions about the everyday running of the Community being discussed by all the Sisters rather than being decided by the Reverend Mother. Similarly, I encouraged the Sisters to discuss their different sense of calling and follow where they thought God wanted them to go. So one of our Sisters trained to be a reflexologist, one started working in a cake shop making the most fabulously decorated cakes, one visited the elderly in a residential home and another started working in interfaith community relations. God can be expressed in whatever we do and whatever talents He has given us. And yes, as well as being the Mother Superior, I am now spiritual director to more than 20 people, as are several of the Sisters.

Then on the eve of the Millennium we all came down with the flu. The Chaplain arrived with a jeroboam of champagne. We were supposed to be having a special midnight service and then a party; instead we had a few sips in the early evening and then all went to bed. It was decided that we needed to look after ourselves a bit better and instituted 'duvet days', where all of us have a couple of free days together after the very busy Christmas and Easter celebrations.

But still occupying our thoughts, prayers, whispered conversations and tense chapter meetings was the fundamental question: what was our real purpose? We had been founded as a nursing community to fill a dire need to look after London's poor. With the foundation of the NHS, this no longer existed. Should we then believe that the Community's work was complete? In the end we did as we always had done: we prayed and we waited. We studied in great depth the essence of the religious life and looked for a new expression of it in a changing world. And gradually a new purpose emerged and continues to grow.

The answer we have come to is that we have to have a willingness to share our life with others, and we should live our life in a way that reflects older examples of the religious life when monasteries and religious houses were generous in sharing their lives. We were fortunate to find ourselves with a large house in a very busy, poor urban area. When we looked around we could see that there was need for a place of prayer and healing, a quiet place in the ever madly dashing world where people can stop and spend time to explore what or indeed Whom their life might be about. Home is a place of safety and refuge, where we welcome in and from which we venture out. One of the things that I loved about Malawi was the hospitality of the people. No matter how poor a family, they would go without food and a bed in order to welcome visitors to their home.

It struck us that in the Mother House we might have a ministry of hospitality. Most importantly, a place where people could experience unconditional, thoughtful love – in the way God loves us and we try to love our fellow human beings, and thus fulfil the ethos of our patron saint, St John the Divine, the apostle of love.

So we have tried to do this by welcoming people from both the Church and the city in which we live. The Sisters form the core Community, and we have our Associates, a band of over 70 friends who are like our extended family, joining the life of the Community as and when they can, and helping to run the house.

One of our first Associates was Sue. She met the Community years ago when she was working with people with HIV and AIDS. Sue had been unimpressed by the lack of concern that the Church had generally shown to the sufferers of this new terrifying illness. That is, until she went to a meeting about AIDS and bumped into two Sisters dressed in blue habits. They smiled at her but Sue glared at them and turned her back. But she bumped into them again at the next meeting, and when still smiling, they invited her to come and talk to them where they were living in Vauxhall, she thought she should give them a chance. Sue was amazed to find four very hard-working Sisters and a house full of love, laughter, and genuine compassion for people living and dying with AIDS. We challenged all her preconceptions about the Church, especially nuns!

The Sisters further won her over when they agreed to take part in an event for World Aids Day, handing out condoms on the street and being photographed by the world's press. In her indomitable way Sister Alice, now well past retirement age, was filmed handing out condoms, telling the reporters: 'We are here because we are human beings caring for other human beings. We believe in the whole ministry of healing and we don't discriminate against anyone.'

After that Sue regularly started to visit the London House and seeing, in a practical way, faith and love at work in the House had something of a conversion and started to build a relationship with God. She has remained a faithful visiting Associate of our community.

We also have our Alongsiders, who come and live with us sometimes for a year or so, fully participating in the life of the Community. People come when they have reached a point in their lives where they have a significant issue that needs to be addressed. Betty arrived at the Mother House at a time of extreme crisis: she was only 25 but her husband had suddenly died. She was a person with major social problems. Every other door had been closed to her, but Betty stayed with us for two and a half years. We listened to Betty and showed her love, but we also kept her busy helping round the house. At first she felt the warmth of just our love, then she began to see our love as something of a reflection of God's love and then began to sense and explore God's love for herself again. It was with huge rejoicing that we held Betty's Confirmation in our chapel. Eventually she felt strong enough to move into her own flat and is now training to work in the Church.

Betty comes back regularly. We are her family now and it has been a huge privilege to be able to help her on her journey.

We also have many visitors, especially the local clergy, who join us for days of reflection, prayer or to study. We host retreats and and study days for individuals and groups. We are still nursing, but nursing souls. It's not always easy: it means we are a family who always have guests at our table. It can be difficult when we are feeling vulnerable and not always welcoming, but this is our challenge. We are born into a world with others, and the face of the other makes a demand on us, a demand that God requires us to answer with hospitality.

In the last two decades we have changed out of all recognition. These are exciting times and yes, it sometimes feels risky, but I think we have found the way that God is leading our Community in the twenty-first century.

In 1998 we celebrated our 150th anniversary with a special service in Birmingham Cathedral. This was a big event for us and terribly exciting, with over 600 people coming from all over the country, some of whom we hadn't seen for years. It was an opportunity to give public thanks for all that had been, for all that is and for all that is to come. With this in mind we decided that we should all have smart new dresses for the occasion.

Our former Reverend Mother, Sarah Grace, had spent the last seven years in happy retirement with us, as a much-loved elder member of the Community. She had been very supportive to me. A few months after I took over from her, she whispered: 'You know I've been watching you, and you've smiled more times in the last 15 weeks than I smiled in the past 15 years. I wish I'd smiled more.' (At which point she *did* smile, somewhat wistfully.)

As the day for our celebration approached we asked her whether she would like us to make her a new dress too.

'Oh no, it would be a waste! I won't wear it again,' she said.

A week after the ceremony, sitting up in her armchair peacefully listening to Radio 4, Sister Sarah Grace died. We buried her ashes in the garden of the Mother House. We missed her greatly, but we were also able to rejoice that she had lived such a full life, with her work joyfully complete.

EPILOGUE

The world has changed out of all recognition since the day in 1957 when I undressed Old Sue and had a vision of myself dressed in a nun's habit. The East End is no longer full of dock workers and big extended families. The insular community, where it might still be an adventure to go to Whitechapel, is long gone. The population is more global and transient. There is poverty but it's a different kind of poverty, less evenly spread; some places are even fashionable, attracting a new kind of wealthier resident, who would never have set foot anywhere near the East End in our day. But I still feel a sense of loss for the wonderful spirit and strong communities that shared their loos and their lives in the years that I worked there.

The work of a midwife has perhaps changed less obviously. In the end, there are only so many ways a baby can be brought into the world. But there has been a shift to a greater emphasis on the theory rather than the practical, to medical intervention and a greater involvement by doctors. Of course the break-up of communities and midwives living in the community has also meant that those precious relationships that we had with our mothers in the district, like Bertha and Jackie Drake, where we knew them and they knew and trusted us, have gone. I think it is a loss, but perhaps inevitable in a world where these kinds of communities have all but disappeared.

But for me the greatest change has been in the lives of the Sisters since the day I travelled up the drive to the Mother House for the first time in 1958, with Sister Clemence crashing into the rhododendrons in the old yellow Morris Minor. When I look back at the long knickers, haircuts, censored reading and formal names to give just a few examples, it's hard to believe those days ever existed. The Community has changed so much, so quickly, that on the surface it's almost unrecognisable.

One of the most striking changes is how the Community is now made up not just of a group of Sisters, but a dynamic group of Associates, Alongsiders and visitors who share our life. Yet underneath I believe the core values, the really important things, most of all the centrality of love and care that is symbolised by our patron, St John the Divine, remain.

However, it has become apparent that there is one thing that still poses a question mark over the future of the Community. While we have our mission which we are confident is a good and God-given one; in order to carry it through in the long term we need more Sisters. There is a core of six of us, together with our new novice, Kim. After Marie-Louise joined us we had no new recruits for ten years, until Eleanor wrote asking to come and stay. She was very young, only 18, and her parents wanted to come with her. Well, we saw no problem in having them but we made it clear to both Eleanor and her parents that we would not consider letting her join us until she was older and had completed her nurse's training.

Eleanor was very persistent. Like so many of us she did not come from a religious family, but through a friend had joined a church choir, and one day during a sermon had received a very strong message that she should become a nun. She also wanted to be a nurse so we suggested she should go and train and at the end of that, if she still thought she might like to join us, she could come back and talk to us. Well, that's exactly what she did. And two years later we went on holiday to the Lake District with another young lady who thought she might have a calling. We had a very jolly time and while climbing a mountain, Eleanor had a strong sense that the time was right to join the Community.

The other lady went to live with our Community in Vauxhall, met a local GP and went off and married! But Eleanor stayed with us and eventually took her life vows in the late 1980s. We were all concerned that she was so much younger than the rest of us – her nearest Sister in age was 20 years older. But we believed that eventually someone would join who was closer to Eleanor's age. Now Eleanor is 50 and we are still waiting.

One reason for this, I believe, is the fact that today there are so many opportunities for women that didn't exist before, not least to become priests. That is a great thing; we have supported women priests all the way, and we pray that women will be allowed to become bishops. But it seems to have pushed into the background other opportunities there may be in the Church for women to pursue a life primarily dedicated to God. However we did start to get enquiries from women who had grown-up children and who were now divorced and interested in dedicating their lives to God.

After much prayer we decided that we should open the way for women who had been married to become Sisters too. Laura came and spent some time with us, stayed, and has now taken her life vows. Her children and grandchildren regularly come and visit and are a wonderful addition to the Community. We also have a novice, Kim, who is doing great interfaithwork in the local community, and her family is also very welcome.

So just as I did as a young novice, every day I pray that there will be women and men who will hear God call them to journey with us. I feel privileged to have had the opportunity to live a life dedicated to responding to others, with love. Now I believe my final vocation is to ensure that when those in need knock at our door there will always be someone to welcome them. In our busy, competitive, individualistic and generally materialistic world, there is a greater need for places offering hospitality and the love of God. So, as old Sister Martha said in the 1920s when the Community was made up of only five elderly Sisters, 'We go on!'

ACKNOWLEDGEMENTS

The Community of St John the Divine would like to thank Helen Batten for the hours of work she has spent both in interviewing the Sisters and in the writing of the book.

As a Community, we would like to dedicate this book to all the Sisters who have gone before us since 1848, for their vision of living the religious life and their pioneering work in both nursing and midwifery.

ABOUT THE SISTERS OF
ST JOHN THE DIVINE

The Community of St John the Divine is a small Anglican community of nuns founded in 1848 in order to bring a better standard of nursing to our hospitals. Much of the Sisters' work took place in the East End and focused on the poor. It is this work that came to the attention of the general public due to Jennifer Worth's books, including *Call the Midwife*, and the TV series of the same name.

Today the Sisters live and work in Birmingham. The ethos of the Community has always concentrated on health and healing, but now it embraces all aspects of health, healing, pastoral care and reconciliation in their widest context. Their website is www.csjd.org.uk.

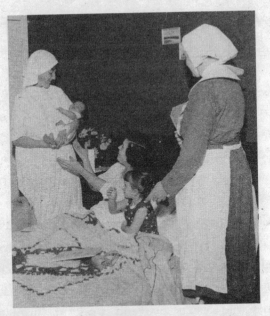

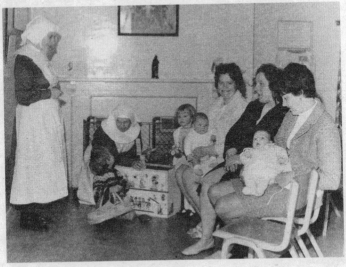

*Nursing and midwifery in the East End
and Deptford in the mid-twentieth century*

*Two Sisters in
about 1850*

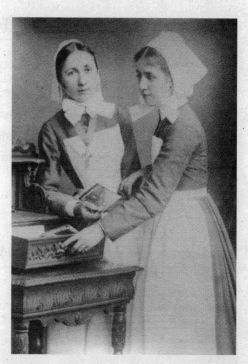

The Sisters today

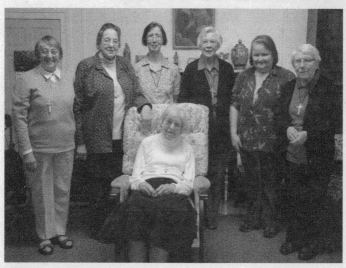

ABOUT THE AUTHOR

Helen Batten studied history at Cambridge and then journalism at Cardiff University. She went on to become a producer and director at the BBC and now works as a writer and a psychotherapist. She lives in West London with her three daughters.

BIBLIOGRAPHY

Cartwright, Dr. F. *The Story of the Community of the Nursing Sisters of St. John the Divine*. King's College Hospital: 1968

Chittister, Joan, OSB. *Wisdom Distilled from the Daily. Living the Rule of St. Benedict Today*. HarperCollins, New York: 1990

Godden, Judith, & Helmstadter, Carol. *Nursing Before Nightingale, 1815–1899, (The History of Medicine in Context)*. Ashgate: 2011

Guenther, Margaret. *Holy Listening, The Art of Spiritual Direction*. Darton, Longman and Todd, London: 1993

Moore, Judith. *A Zeal for Responsibility – The Struggle for Professional Nursing in Victorian England, 1868–1883*. Athens, University of Georgia: 1988